HELP
for your
Aching Back!

HELP
for your
Aching Back!

By

Harvey P. Kopell, M. D.
and
Nancy C. Kester, M. D.

Published in Association with
PARADE MAGAZINE

GROSSET & DUNLAP

Publishers   **New York**

Introduction

BERNARD BARUCH once said, "I am interested in physical medicine because my father was, I am interested in rehabilitation because I believe in it, and I am interested in arthritis because I've got it." I personally can discuss low back pain poignantly and achingly because I've got it.

Reading the chapter on trauma vividly recalls the lean bay horse that somersaulted over a jump more than twenty years ago with me somersaulting over the horse on the hard-packed Missouri clay and gives me an excruciating pain in the back just to remember it.

Drs. Kopell and Kester have done a masterful job in discussing and putting in perspective the problems of the aching back, a condition causing more discomfort, loss of time from work and disability than any other. Their remarks on mores in various countries throughout the world gives interesting insight as to cause and frequency. Fashions through the years, from corsets to modern dancing, also have played their part in both causing and aggravating this painful curse of our time.

The illustrations in the book are mechanically and mathematically ingenious. They are informative not only to the layman but to the physician, both the generalist and the specialist. The discussion on diagnostic and surgical procedures, physical therapy and other therapeutic procedures are straightforward as to their indication and contra-indication and are put in perspective with a common-sense approach. The sections on rest, sleep, sports and even sex are frankly discussed and make an important contribution.

The authors have made a real contribution to the understanding and common-sense therapeutic approach to the "aching back." It makes interesting and informative reading both to the sufferer and the practitioner.

HOWARD A. RUSK, M.D.

Contents

1

The Back Problem

IF A SITUATION lasts long enough it will produce its own words and even full phrases. World War II had its share. Such expressions as "G.I.," "Snafu," "Kilroy was here," and "Oh, my aching back," are remnants of the conflict. For our purpose, the last—"Oh, my aching back"—is most interesting. Its origin must be based on the fact that the back played an important part in many G.I.s' thinking. The long life of the expression testifies to its popular application. The use of the term as an exclamation also reveals that emotional stress might work out as a back disability.

The war can be used for another illustration which took place one night in the darkened ward of a general hospital. A group of badly wounded men had just been evacuated from the Battle of the Bulge. For the most part they were happy to be away from the front and through with traveling for a while. Some had both arms in a cast, some were in casts from the waist on down. All in this shipment had been seriously wounded. It was quiet; then, suddenly, from a dark back corner of the ward came a frantic call: "Medic! Medic! I'm in agony!" The medical officer went back to look at the man's tag. The patient who was in such severe distress had a back condition. Just why his problem should have required such urgent medical attention over and beyond the men with severe open wounds is one of the peculiarities of the backache with which we will try to deal.

Another point in the general consideration of the back problem is the variety of back treatment available. Any person with back trouble can, within a short space of time, meet up with many well-meaning opinions as to different types of treatment. The treatment offered ranges from manipulation through medicine, rest and surgery. If the advice is examined it will be seen that each has its success and failures, and often one's success is based on another's failure. The conclusions that can be drawn are:

1. All back aches are not the same. Each group requires its own form of treatment.
2. Different individuals respond to different forms of treatment.
3. Perhaps after a certain period of time any different form of treatment will work.

The expression, "Oh, my aching back," is American. This raises the point of whether all countries have the same back problem. The answer is difficult, as worthwhile figures that lend themselves to statistical analysis are hard to find. There can be many social and economic factors that determine the importance of a bad back in a particular country. A doctor from India has said that the bad back, either acute or chronic, was a minor problem in his country. His analysis of the factors that worked against the occurrence of bad backs was interesting.

1. Very few Indian people sleep on soft beds. A firm, flat sleeping surface gives better rest for the low back.
2. The Indian worker does hard physical labor in a fairly continuous fashion. It was the doctor's belief that American workers do heavy bursts of hard physical labor with long pauses in between. The pause allows so much relaxation of muscles that,

when the next burst of activity calls for a properly concerted muscular activity pattern, individual muscles are not ready for it. The pattern for proper muscular interplay for work activity is off.

3. The individual Indian worker tries to keep sudden efforts within his tolerance by the use of assistance. He had noted that when a porter had to carry a heavy piece of luggage he would get a friend to help put it on his back and then help him balance it so that it could be carried without the extra stress of trying to get it in balance. He would not attempt to place it on his back by just his own efforts.

4. Most Indian people do not wear constricting shoes. The better foot and toe motions make for a better gait. This in turn makes for better, more efficient alignment on the part of the hip, back and trunk musculature. Their walking posture is better than that of the shoe wearer.

5. Of course, there is the factor which was not gone into in great detail—the difference of compensation for injury and the ease of securing medical attention in the two countries.

The discussion of these factors won't help directly with our own back conditions but it can furnish us with some insight into the problem. We can deduce from the above that maintaining the back musculature in good condition and avoiding sudden overwhelming stress is important to prevent trouble. The tendency towards an increasing push-button existence must inevitably lead to greater weakening of not only the back but the entire muscular system. And always it must be remembered that it is just not that a specific muscle gets weak through lack of use, but that patterns of muscle activity get ragged and uneven if they are not reinforced by activity.

An example of this is to be found in an "efficiency" kitchen. In one of these, the worker does not have to move around very much. Almost everything can be reached, stretched for, or bent for from one spot. Now take the same worker and put her in a less efficient kitchen with more space. She has to walk to get ingredients, pots, or water. At the end of a fixed period, say two hours, the worker in the less efficient kitchen will have fewer aches and sore muscles, and perhaps, too, be less prone to backaches. The worker in the efficiency kitchen will be more tired, because muscles and ligaments stand movement more easily than continued contraction for maintenance of position.

The extra demands of activity—walking, full unobstructed reaching—serve also to relieve tensions and are important as to how much fatigue the person feels after a period of work. The exact nature of fatigue or tiredness is still not clearly understood. The reason is that the feeling is not just the effect of physical effort. The mind and the emotions are also involved in how tired one feels.

One of the effects of fatigue that is of major concern in the back problem is the tendency to accidents. The accidents that can occur because of fatigue are not only external—stumbling over objects, for example—but internal as well—pulled muscles, strained ligaments, and the like—caused by errors of judgment in movement. This does not have to be on a conscious level but usually occurs as a result of ragged patterning of muscular activity—poor interplay of muscle actions—either in timing or the force exerted.

2

Spine Fashions

THE BACKACHE HAS been around for a long time. People have had lumbago and sciatica for many years. Throughout its long history the ideas about origin and treatment of backache have changed. Sixty or seventy years ago it was believed that sciatica was caused chiefly by an inflammation of the sciatic nerve. Now we recognize that the word "sciatica" is purely a descriptive term, a word like "rash." The word "rash" describes a skin condition, it does not imply that the skin discoloration or change of texture has been caused by a specific disease. A rash can be caused by many things, from an allergy to measles. Sciatica means that there is pain that starts in the buttock and runs down the back of the leg, even down to the toes. It can be caused by a herniated disc pressing on a nerve root, an inflammation of any portion of the sciatic nerve or its branches, or even a tumor in the pelvis. The idea that many cases of sciatica are caused by irritation of the roots of the sciatic nerve in their passage out of the spine, as from a slipped disc, is comparatively recent. Up to thirty years ago it was felt that the origin of most back difficulties was in the sacro-iliac joints. The statement "it was felt" means that most responsible treating physicians thought that way. Inflammation, sprains, and subluxa-

13

tions (displacement of the joint surfaces—to a lesser degree than a full dislocation) were thought to be the cause.

To show the progress of medical knowledge with relation to popular understanding, it is only necessary to recall a song of the 1940's, "The South American Way," sung by Bing Crosby and the Andrews Sisters. In the chorus there is a plea to take back the South American Way as it is causing the singers' sacro-iliac to go out of whack. Aside from fulfilling a need for a rhyme, the statement implied that everyone knew what the sacro-iliac was and that painful disability can result from an improper relationship in that region. From the standpoint of the spread of medical opinion to the people, at the time the song was popular the sacro-iliac joint was on its way to slipping away to obscurity. The slipped disc, the lumbo-sacral joint, was rising as a major source of low back difficulty. Now the general public knows about such things as a slipped or herniated disc, spine fusions and myelograms. The proof of the spread of this knowledge can be found in catalogs of one of the most widely known mail order houses. Through the catalog it is possible to buy a support that not only will help a painful back but also "help to prevent a slipped disc." It is taken for granted that the general public knows how bad a slipped disc can be. Nowadays the term sacro-iliac sprain is only used on rare occasions. As far as we are concerned, the term has to be called forth when dealing with a patient who was once up on his medical terminology but who has not kept up, or with insurance personnel still using the forms of yesteryear.

The term "lumbago," once very popular, is now out of fashion. It referred to pain in the lumbar region. It once had meaning as a cause, but as diagnostic skill improved, it also came to be a purely descriptive word. It was seen to be an effect, not a cause. It may be that part of its fall from grace as a good descriptive word is that it seems, just from the standpoint of a word, to lack

14

force. Keeping pace with its fading away was the declining use of the medicated plaster as a cure for the bad back, although it still sells in rural areas.

There have been changes in outlook and treatment of the bad back. This has been caused by the inadequacy of many of the older treatments to take care of serious back conditions. In some of the milder varieties of a back condition, the passage of time relieved the condition. But with the increasing value of time and the desire for more rapid and definitive rehabilitation of the disabled, the need has come about for better initial evaluation of the condition and better results from proposed treatment. For this it is necessary to have some appreciation of back structure and function.

3

Form and Structure
of the Back

THE ACTION AND the malfunction of the back cannot be appreciated properly or dealt with usefully if just one element, spine or disc, is considered to the exclusion of the rest of the system. The back consists of fixed, active and passive structures. The fixed structures are the bones, called the vertebrae, and, to a great extent, the connecting ligaments. Ligaments are the fibrous structures (like gristle) that tie bones together.

The active structures are the muscles and their tendons. The tendons are fibrous structures—again like gristle—that transmit the power of the muscle to the bone. Most spinal muscles have very little tendonous portion; they tend to insert directly onto the bone. When a chop, such as a lamp chop, is eaten, the muscle mass that is the edible portion is one of the spinal muscles. It will be seen in most cuts to attach on the bone. Chops are meat that is a cut across the spinal muscles of the animal.

The passive structures are the elements such as the intervertebral disc which can be extruded or pushed out of place and in so doing cause pressure on another passive structure, the nerve root. When this happens the signs and symptoms of a herniated (commonly called "slipped") disc occur. Ligaments are the fibrous material

16

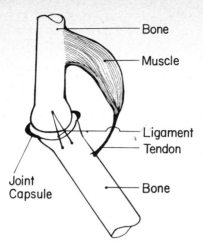

Figure 1.   The elements of a joint.

that tie one bone to another. A ligament begins and ends on a bone. Although it can exert an elastic tension, it cannot actively contract like a muscle.

The role of these structures in the function of the spine as a whole must be considered. The lumbar spine connects the lower portions of the body to the upper. It maintains the upper part of the body erect on the lower portion. It is the lumbar spine apparatus that enables the man to

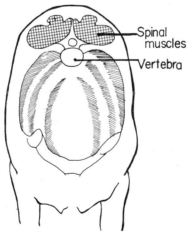

Figure 2.   Cross-section of a steer, showing the spinal muscles (steak).

stand erect and to move the upper portion of his body with relation to his lower limbs. Not only does the spine maintain a posture but it participates in a change of posture. The spine contains and protects a canal through which pass the nerves that carry the messages of the upper nervous system to and from the lower portion of the body. The flexibility of the spine, its ability to move in more than one plane, or swivel, gives it a universal

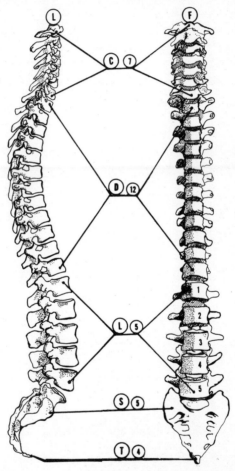

Figure 3. Side and front view of vertebral column. C—cervical vertebrae; D—dorsal or thoracic vertebrae; L—lumbar vertebrae; S—sacral vertebrae (fused); T—coccyx or coccygeal vertebrae.

joint action. This smooths out the transmission of *propulsive* force to the neck and head so the neck and head can be carried without the jolting that walking or running would produce.

It is now necessary to look at the spine more closely. It is divided into a number of regions. From the top down: the cervical (neck); thoracic or dorsal (region behind chest); lumbar; sacral (portion that joins with the pelvis); and coccygeal (the very end of the spine). Coccygeal is the adjective, coccyx is the noun. Compound or hyphenated words are often used to describe the junction of two portions; for example, cervico-thoracic (or cervico-dorsal), thoraco-lumbar (or dorso-lumbar), lumbo-sacral (or sacro-coccygeal) regions. These regions are important, since often the effects of trauma concentrate here and cause more injury at these junction regions.

The bone unit that is the basis of the vertebral column is the vertebra. And although each vertebra is a little different from its neighbor, they have certain common features. In its most abstract form it consists of two

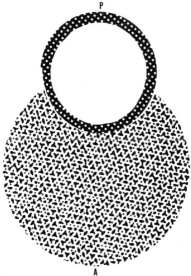

Figure 4. Abstract diagram of a vertebra, from above. P—back; A—front.

circles, one a ring of bone, the other a solid cylinder of bone. The ring presses into the cylinder. When the vertebrae are stacked one on top of each other, the rings form a tube which contains and protects the spinal cord. The spinal cord connects the parts of the body to each other and to the brain. The spinal cord sends and receives its information out of the spinal canal through nerve roots.

The vertebrae are connected to each other by joints. There are three joint surfaces for each neighbor, so that each vertebra has six joint surfaces—three for the one above, three for the one below. The solid cylinder portion of the vertebra is called the body. The bodies of neighboring vertebrae are tied together by ligaments and a ring of fibrous tissues which surrounds the intervertebral disc. This joint here is body-intervertebral disc-body. Next we have the spinal joints, one on each side. which meet up with the joints of the neighbor. It will be seen from the diagram that there are holes produced when one vertebra joins up with the other through which the nerve roots come. Each hole is known as a foramen. The nerve roots pass through the foramen. Here in this bony opening which will not yield to pressure, they can easily be injured by anything pressing against the ring.

The amount of motion that can take place between the vertebrae differs in different portions of the spine. The cervical and lumbar regions move relatively freely. They can be moved passively by an outside force and they can be moved voluntarily without specific training.

The thoracic vertebrae are connected to the ribs, which, in turn, are connected to a fairly rigid piece of bone, the sternum (or breast bone). Therefore, the thoracic vertebrae have a small range of motion with relation to each other.

The five vertebrae that form the sacrum are normally fused together into one mass. This mass is joined to the pelvis on either side by the sacro-iliac joints. The sacrum forms the back wall of the pelvic region.

Each section of the spinal column has a characteristic

20

sweeping curve in the adult. At birth and very early age the curve is different. The whole spine is flexed into a C-shaped curve which opens forward. The wave-shaped curves in the adult spine would seem to have the purpose of increasing the flexibility of the spine as a whole. The curves are important, for if we imagine the spine as a fixed tube in the adult, then every jolt in walking, running or jumping would be transmitted up that straight line to the skull. Repeated concussions would soon come about from any type of physical activity. The give in the curves, possible through the ligaments that bind the vertebrae together and the intervertebral discs, softens the forces that are transmitted upward. (See Figure 3.)

There is no inherent stability of the vertebrae. They cannot be piled one on top of the other like building blocks or poker chips. The column will fall down. Adjacent bones throughout the body are connected by ligaments. These are tough fibrous strands or bundles familiar to meat eaters as gristle. If the vertebrae are bound together in a normal fashion by their ligaments, the cervical and lumbar portions will still not remain upright. This requires muscular action. (The fused sacrum and the thoracic spine, maintained by the ribs and sternum, will hold a vertical position.) The need for muscular action to maintain the upright position is easily seen in the fact that an unconscious person slumps down.

It may seem strange that a long railway trip should be so fatiguing when the passenger is constantly seated. The reason is that the constant jolting and jerking of the train would throw him off balance if active muscular action were not used to right himself back to the erect position. Also the constant righting efforts in a seated position, where there is a mechanical disadvantage, demands greater effort on the part of the trunk musculature.

The ligaments that run between the vertebrae bind them together. They act as checks to prevent too much motion. They help to stabilize the point. The ring-shaped ligament that runs between two vertebral bodies has a special function—it forms a ring that holds the intervertebral disc in place. The ligament is called the annular ligament (from annulus: ring). When the annular ligament tears, the disc substance can come out. The disc is of a thick gelatinous consistency in its normal state. It is a little softer than a gelatin dessert that has been in a refrigerator too long. If the disc herniates (common terminology: slips out) it can press on nerve roots, to give the signs and symptoms of a disc syndrome. This will be discussed in greater detail later.

The annular ligament is made up of alternating layers of fibrous tissue. A good analogy for this is the Chinese finger trap. As with the Chinese finger trap certain motions of the ligament can damage the fibers. Other motions can be performed without impairing the strength of the fibers. If the finger trap is subject to alternate shearing forces or too much twisting, then the fibers begin to fray.

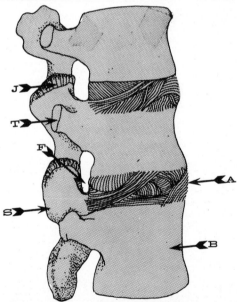

Figure 5. Side view of vertebrae. A—annulus fibrosus (note criss-cross overlap of fibres); B—vertebral body; F—intervertebral foramen; J—intervertebral joint; T—transverse process; S—spinous process.

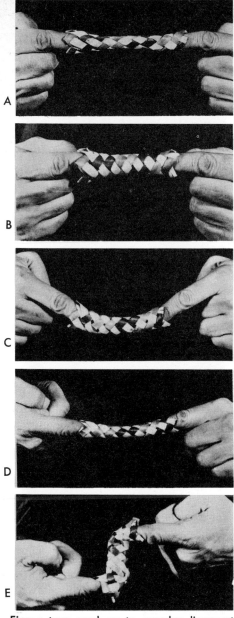

Figure 6. Finger trap analogy to annular ligament. A—tension; B—compression; C—angulation; D—twisting (torsion); E—shearing.

While thousands and thousands of cycles of compression and extension, bending, and perhaps fewer on twisting can be performed without damage to the fibers, only a few hundred cycles of shearing motion will cause the fibers to start fraying. To transpose this analogy to the body, when two vertebrae move with relation to each other in a normal manner, the annular ligament tends to remain intact. When an external force overcomes ligament and muscular protection or improper muscular action causes unnatural motion such as shearing, then the annulus can wear thin and tear. This will permit the disc to bulge out.

It is important to see how the muscles act on the spine. Here, too, an analogy may be helpful in understanding the mechanics of the system. Suppose two firemen are trying to position a ladder against a building. The plan is for Fireman A to walk under the ladder increasing its upward elevation as he walks. But to accomplish this it is necessary that fireman B place his feet against the bottom of the ladder. If he does not stabilize that end—

Figure 7.   Firemen raising a ladder.

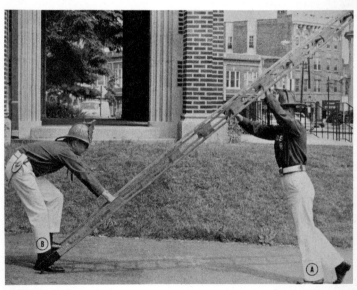

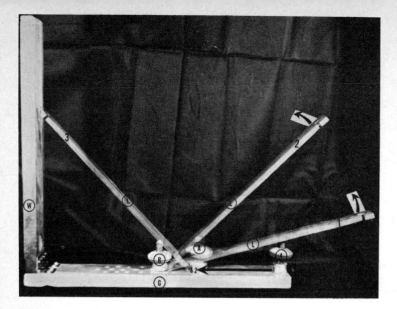

Figure 8. Fireman (A) moves from 1 to 2 and 3 to raise ladder (L) from 1 to 3 against the wall (W). Fireman (B) establishes fulcrum by pegging it in a hole in the ground (G).

establish a fulcrum—the work of Fireman A will just shove it forward. To raise the ladder successfully we need a prime mover—Fireman A—and a stable hinge, pivot or fulcrum point—Fireman B. In the body too, for most joints to move, we need not only a prime mover (the major muscle that moves the joint), but also some means of maintaining the joint, the pivot point of motion. The joint stabilization mechanism may be chiefly bone, as in the elbow; muscles, as in the shoulder; or a combination of muscles and ligaments, as in the knee.

To further illustrate the point of fulcrum establishment, the model shown in Figure 8 was prepared. Fireman B is able to maintain his fulcrum point because a peg is inserted into a hole in the ground board. Fireman A, by moving forward, causes the ladder to rise.

But this illustration is faulty in one respect: Muscles don't push, they pull. Their active force comes from a contraction. To show this, we take away Fireman A, who was pushing forward, and substitute a string that pulls the end of the ladder upward. And here a new term is

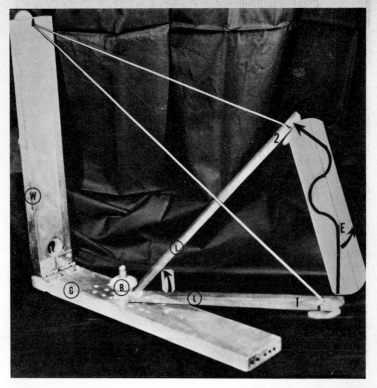

Figure 9. String (prime mover) picks up ladder (L) from 1 to 2 against pivot (B). Note erratic course (E) taken by ladder.

introduced: the prime mover. This is the muscle that is chiefly responsible for the final act. In the mechanical example shown here, the string is the prime mover. It causes the end of the ladder to move upward, pivoting at the point maintained by Fireman B.

Now if the string is pulled upward an unusual event occurs: The ladder moves wildly or uncontrollably out of the plane in which it is supposed to move. The multiple exposure technique used in Figure 9 shows the instability at the pivot point. There is need for some means of fulcrum stabilization. To do this, two posts are set up on either side of the ladder. These prevent the unwanted sideways swinging. The new, now-useful controlled motion is shown in the multiple exposures of Figure 11. It can be seen that there are two jobs to be

26

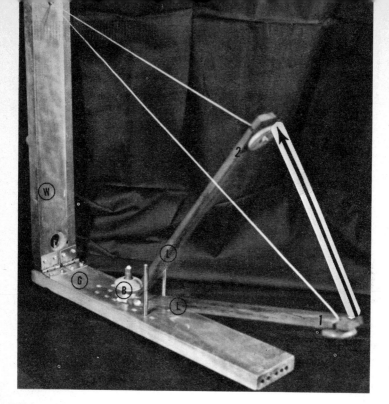

Figure 10. String (prime mover) picks up end of ladder (L) from 1 to 2; other end of ladder is stabilized against pivot point (B) by the two vertical rods. Note smooth path taken by ladder as compared with that in Figure 9.

done at the pivot region. The first is to set up the point at which the pivoting occurs; the second is to maintain stability at the point of motion. When you try to open a door that has two hinges, and the screws that hold the hinge plates to the door are loose, you will find that a great deal of force will be necessary. The hinges provide a pivot, but if the hinges are loose you have to apply extra force beyond opening the door to maintain the pivot point.

The elements that form a functioning joint, not only in the spine but elsewhere in the body, can now be understood. These elements are:

1. a pivot point, which includes joint surfaces,

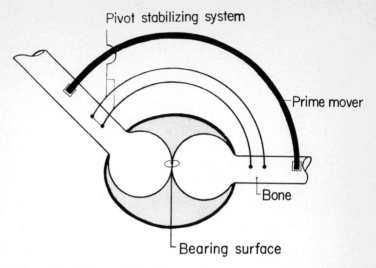

Figure 11. Elements of a joint.

2. a means of stabilizing the pivot,
3. the prime mover.

Two of these elements, the prime mover and the pivot point or joint surfaces, are easily understood.

The prime movers must be able to contract properly; they must respond in time with the right amount of force. At the point where the two limbs of the joint pivot, the bearing surfaces must be smooth and offer no impediment to motion. Think of the difference in closing a door with a rusty hinge as compared to one with a smooth, well-oiled hinge. In most cases of pivoting joints the bearing surfaces are held together within a small sack. The sack covering is called the joint capsule. The lining of the capsule is called the synovium. Inside the capsule there is a small amount of fluid, the synovial fluid. This fluid can be considered a lubricating medium.

The action of the pivot stabilizing mechanism is fundamental to the proper action of the joint. Without stabilization the action of the prime movers would soon disrupt the joint. The pivot or fulcrum is stabilized by bone in some joints, ligaments in others, and by small muscles in most of the joints that carry a heavy load. The bulk of these stabilizing muscles are called synergists. The meaning of that word is "to work with." The synergists work with the prime movers. The action of the synergists must be appropriate for the action of the prime movers. If the synergists' force is too little or too late, the joint will not be properly stabilized for a heavy load. If the synergists contract too hard and too soon they might "freeze" the joint. The mechanics describe a similar situation with the term "a seized bearing." If the prime movers work against the "seized" joint they will be overstrained.

These points can now be tied together with relation to a functional model of the spine.

Figure 12 consists of two illustrations. One is a vertebra as normally seen, the second is a line drawing which enables an understanding of function without becoming involved in anatomical detail.

1 is the vertebral body.
2 is the neural arch.
3 is the spinous process.

Figure 12a. Vertebra viewed from back.

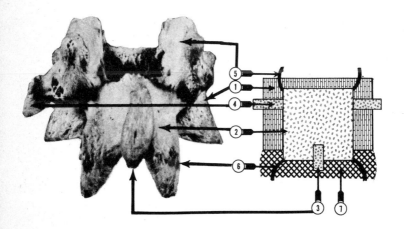

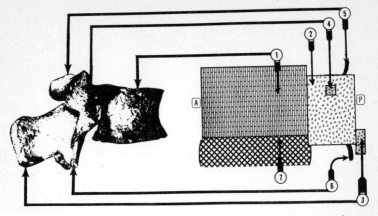

Figure 12b. Vertebra viwed from side (lateral view). A—front; P—back.

4 is the transverse process. Muscles attach to both the transverse and spinous processes.

5 is the upper joints.

6 is the lower joints

7 is the intervertebral disc surrounded by the annular ligament

The nerve roots and the foramen through which they pass will be shown later. These points are often seen better in one view than in the other.

In Figure 13, two vertebrae are joined· Now the capsule is shown by the enclosure 8, around the joints. The small muscles are shown as bands running from attachment points on the spinous and transverse processes. The muscles that run from one vertebra to another serve to stabilize the joint for motion.

Some of the small muscles skip one or more vertebrae and may attach over the span of more than one. These muscles serve to stabilize one group of vertebrae against another group, so that each of the two groups forms a lever arm. Of course, this is an ultra-abstraction since, although there is a major pivot point for one motion at one space, all the vertebrae in one section participate in

30

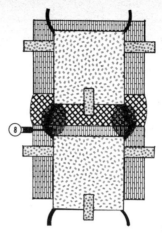

Figure 13a. Back view of two vertebrae joined together. (8) is joint surrounded by capsule.

Figure 13b. Side view of two vertebrae joined together. A—front; P—back; F—foramen; black area is nerve root.

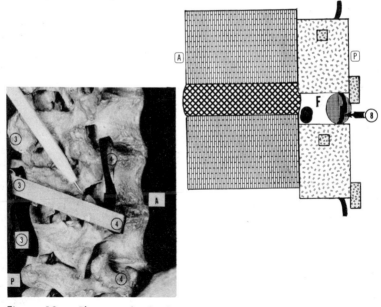

Figure 13c. Photograph of side view of spine with fulcrum stabilizing system represented by tapes. A—front; P—back; 3—spinous process; 4—transverse process. The pen points to the joint.

the motion. This makes for a supple spine. But the figure illustrates the work of the multi-level muscles.

For the next components we can use Figure 19a (page 51) to show the major prime movers (12). This shows the sacrum, 10, and the pelvis, 11. The line drawing is out of proportion but it does not interfere with the demonstration. The place where the lumbar vertebrae join the sacrum is called the lumbo-sacral junction. And the place where the sacrum is connected to the pelvis is called the sacro-iliac joint; there is one on each side.

The prime movers are designated as 12. Although there are actually more, just these shown will serve. To put in more would add too much complexity to the diagram.

Figure 13c is a photograph of a spine with strips of tape used to simulate the fulcrum stabilization system. The pointer is directed to the joint on which the small muscles stabilize.

Another diagram is suggested by the two prime mover muscles—the stays on a sloop (Figure 14). The mast guy lines maintain the mast upright. This is the same type of system that enables the living spine to maintain a position and even an upright posture. The spinal system is very well muscled in four-legged animals and even those without legs. The system acts to maintain a fixed axial base against which the more removed parts, the limbs, can move.

Throughout this discussion the emphasis has been on muscle activity. There is little that the individual can do himself to alter the fixed elements (bone) of the spine, but he can change the active elements (muscles). In so doing, in time, he can influence the passive elements (ligaments and discs). The change in muscular action is not just a change in strength. Undoubtedly of greater importance is the relationship of the action of one muscle to another. The point of muscular interplay or timing can be noted in the most casual glance at the athletic scene. In any sport the excellence of an athlete cannot be judged by looking at his muscular development or measuring the

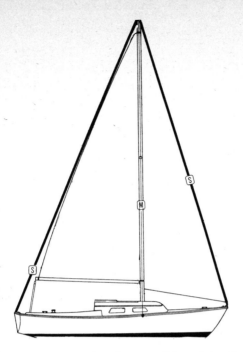

Figure 14. Stays (S) maintain the mast (M) upright. Only one side stay is shown against the mast.

strength of any individual muscle. Rather it is the pattern of muscular activity that is most important—how the action of one dovetails into another. After all, the exact physical attributes of Babe Ruth, Joe DiMaggio, and Willie Mays do not match. There are many baseball players who have the same size shoulders or arms who are not champion hitters.

I once observed a life guard at a summer resort. He was built well. Each of his muscles stood out in anatomical purity. He expressed his awareness of his appearance by referring to himself as the "Greek God." But he could hardly run; he could not scale a shell as well as a twelve-year-old, and his swimming was testimony to the political basis of his appointment to the job. Although he was very strong, he was an exposition of the term "muscle bound." His individual muscles were strong; the interplay of muscular action was weak.

When we speak of athletes, we realize that there is an interrelationship between muscle form and use. The legs of a ballet dancer are different from those of a swimmer. There is a difference in muscle shape between the arms of a boxer and a soccer player. But any sport, including weight lifting, requires the proper sequence of muscular activity.

4

Disc Herniation

ARMED WITH IDEAS about the structure and the function of the spinal column it is now possible to go on to the subject of the herniated disc. The spinal canal serves as a conduit and a protective enclosure of nerve tissue. The major nerve tissue in the canal is the spinal cord and its prolongation into nerve roots. Although the spinal cord has other independent functions, a major purpose is to carry the nerve fibers to and from the brain, through nerve roots, to the level where they serve their final purpose—either to carry sensation back to the brain, or the impulse to muscles to contract. The nerve fibers leave the spinal cord for each level of the body in bundles that are called nerve roots. Nerve fibers soon leave the nerve roots to travel along with nerve fibers from other roots. The new bundles thus formed finally assume new identities as peripheral nerves. The peripheral nerves roughly maintain their distribution corresponding to the level at which they left the spinal column.

The nerve root is vulnerable to pressure effects as it comes through the foramen. This is the hole formed between two vertebrae that permits the passage of the root. (See Figure 15.)

Figure 16 is a view looking down at the fourth lumbar vertebrae. Everything above that level has been removed.

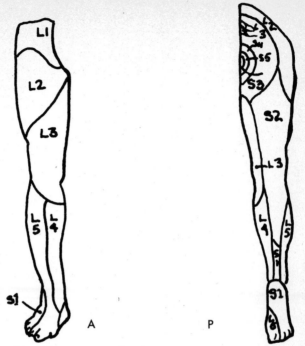

Figure 15. Nerve root distribution. A—front; P—back. These boundaries may vary somewhat in different individuals.

The disc substance is seen lying within the annulus fibrosus—the fibrous ring. The nerve roots are lying free about to enter the foramen. The foramen is no longer a hole but is now a trough, since its top half has been removed.

Figure 16 shows the disc which has broken through a tear in the annulus fibrosus. It is now in a position to compress the nerve root against the hard wall of the foramen.

Pressure on the nerve root will usually cause pain. The muscle supplied by the nerve root will be weak and if the pressure lasts long enough there will be atrophy (wasting). Sensation from the supplied region will diminish and, if the pressure is great enough, it will disappear and the area will become numb.

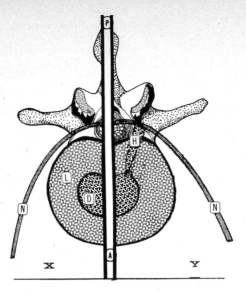

Figure 16. View looking down at vertebra disc, showing relationship of disc (D) to nerve roots (N). X—normal side; Y—herniated disc side; P—back: A—front; L—annular ligament (annulus fibrosus); H—herniated disc.

It was stated above that pain can be produced by pressure on a nerve root. There can be pain in the low back and in the portion of the limb supplied by nerve fibers. To understand this last point, the nerve root should be considered as a telephone wire. (See Figure 17.)

Y is trying to communicate with X. If the wire is cut either at point A or point B, X will not receive the message. If the wires are frayed and the insulation worn thin, then static will be produced. If pressure is made at either point A or point B to fray the wires then the listener at point X will not know (unless he has special instruments) whether the static is coming from point A or point B or even if it originates at Y itself.

If we now transpose this analogy to nerve terms, we let X be the sensing individual and the telephone wire the nerve root extending to skin or muscle which is at Y. The static is equal to pain. If pressure is made on the nerve root in the foramen, point A, pain will be felt in that nerve root projection as though it came from the

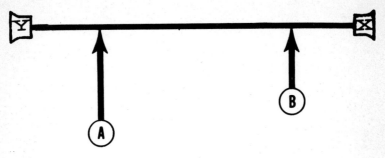

Figure 17. Y is trying to communicate with X.

skin or muscle which is at point B. This occurs even though no nerve irritation takes place at point B.

Nerves, when pinched or squeezed, do not yield information to the individual as to the point where they are pinched. By analysis of the complaints and interpretation of the signs the physician can often draw a conclusion as to the point of disturbance. In many cases, special instruments and techniques are necessary to determine the exact site of the pressure. By analysis of many facts available as to the distribution and intensity of the findings the physician can determine further if the difficulty is in a nerve root or in a peripheral nerve.

Abnormal function of a nerve root will affect a particular region. The most commonly affected roots are in the Lumbar 4 and 5 region. The pain from this level will radiate from the buttock down (sciatic distribution—sciatica). The skin regions noted in the diagram will be affected. Muscles supplied by these roots will be weak and even atrophied. One of the functions of the motor nerve (nerve to a muscle) is to transmit the impulse for the deep tendon reflexes—knee jerk and ankle jerk.

When tendons are sharply jerked—as when struck briskly with a blunt object—an impulse is sent to the spinal cord via the nerve root. An impulse is then returned to the muscle which causes a sharp contraction. There are a number of diseases which can alter this reaction, either causing an exaggerated response, which we term hyperactive, or making it less, or hypoactive. Pressure on a nerve root as from a herniated disc is one of the conditions that can cause anything from hypoactivity to complete absence in the deep tendon reflexes, depending on the level of the pressure.

The L4-L5-S1, or lumbo-sacral, region is emphasized. This is no accidental choice. The majority of low back difficulties occur in this region. The fact can be explained on a physical basis. Whenever a system contains energy in motion, the energy will tend to concentrate or exert most force at the region where there is a change in state. The change in state can be a difference in diameter, a difference in density or a difference in flexibility. There are numerous examples of this in the world around us. The most easily recognizable can be seen in the ordinary electric iron. At the point where the electric cord enters the instrument the manufacturer usually puts a spiral spring sleeve or rubber cuff. Besides the electrical energy,

Figure 18. Electric iron. Note the coil where the wire enters the iron. This spring-like coil helps to dissipate the stress at this region.

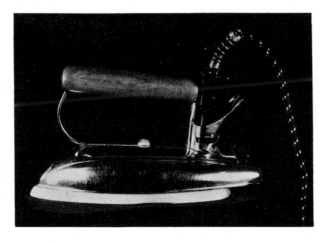

the act of ironing makes the cord contain a great deal of mechanical energy as it moves around. Through experience it has been learned that this energy concentrates at the point where the cord enters the iron. At this point the cord changes from a flexible state to a non-flexible state. The increased amount of energy at this point would soon make the insulation fray and cause the wires inside to break. To guard against this the spring or rubber cuff is used. This spreads the energy over a longer portion of the cord—4 inches instead of 1/40 inch—and makes for a more gradual transition from a freely moveable to the fixed cord state. (Figure 18.)

In the spine the same relationship is present at the lumbo-sacral junction. The sacral vertebrae are normally fused into a single bony mass. The lumbar vertebrae above them are free to move with relation to each other and the sacrum. It is the region in which there is an abrupt change of state in the spinal system; therefore energy accumulates here and exerts more force. Tissues have only a certain amount of tolerance to mechanical force. The tolerance can be exceeded, either all at once or by frequent small amounts over a period of time. The outcome will depend not only on the tissue damage produced by the force but the amount and quality of repair that occurs. The ability to repair depends on many factors—nourishment (food and oxygen available), amount of repeated damage, and other factors such as hormones. The final state can be influenced, too, by how other elements substitute or take over the action of the destroyed or incompletely repaired portions.

The repair of damaged tissues may vary from almost like new to grossly inadequate. The higher we go in the animal scale the less ability there is for complete replacement healing. In the low order amphibians, such as the salamander, a tail or a leg can be removed and the animal is capable of growing a new one. As we go higher in the animal scale the repair abilities become less and less. In the higher forms, tissues are not replaced as well. A tear in muscle, elastic tissue or nerve is more apt to be replaced by a fibrous scar than by the original type. This fact is important in considering the recovery from an injury. If the muscle, either a part of the stabilization system or a prime mover, is torn, the replacement scar does not have the ability to contract or resist force as does the intact muscle. If the scar is not too big, the rest of the muscle bulk can compensate for the deficiency, and, under certain circumstances, other nearby parallel action muscles may substitute their function for the damaged muscle.

A ligament normally contains elastic fibers. It should have a tough type of elasticity. It is somewhat similar to the dense, firm rubber found in an automobile tire. The elastic fibers continue into the bone substance to give a solid attachment of the ligament to the bone. If the ligament is overstretched and the elastic fibers in it are torn, or the entire ligament is ripped across, the repair will be made by fibrous tissue rather than by new elastic fibers. This new fibrous tissue, the scar, does not have the same properties as the original tissue. It cannot take the abuse or wear that the elastic tissue did. It will not give with a sudden force. As it has so little ability to yield, the force may cause another tear and so provide the basis for further fibrosis.

However, replacement fibrosus does not have to remain as such. With time and proper mechanical stimulation (not abuse), the fibrotic region may shrink down and there can be slow growth of the original tissue elements. This is the hope and one of the main goals of the treatment for a chronic low back derangement.

5

Spine Posture

UP TO THIS point attention has been directed to individual elements of the spine. Now we have to put the pieces together and look at the structure as a whole. Posture, or the shape of the structure when the pieces are in place, can determine the strain that the individual elements must put up with. Posture is not only the result of the shape of the individual vertebrae, but also the forces that act on the vertebrae. Some of this is under conscious control; a major portion is involuntary.

The lumbar spine in the adult, viewed from front or back, under normal conditions is straight up and down. There should be no tilt to either side. Viewed from the side there is a complex, S-shaped curve—the S looking backward (Figure 3). If we look at an x-ray of the lateral view, we can see that two lines can be drawn to form an angle—the lumbo-sacral angle. If the angle is small, L5, which is transmitting the weight of the trunk above it, will press directly down on the sacrum, or S1. If the angle is large, then the pressure of the body weight above the level will exert a force that pushes the L5 vertebra forward on S1.

It can be seen that the body weight tends to thrust down in the direction of arrow A and the supporting force tends to push up in the direction of arrow B. The more A moves in the direction of S1 (increasing the lumbo-sacral angle), the more shearing force will occur at the lumbo-sacral junction. It has been shown previously with relation to the ligament (the annulus fibrosis) that shearing force is bad. It is the type of force that puts most strain on the junction, and causes most wear of the fulcrum stabilizing ligaments and muscles.

A number of factors can increase the lumbo-sacral angle. If, for example, the muscles and ligaments that cross the front of the hip joint are tight, the relationship of the pelvis to the lumbar spine is altered, and the lumbo-sacral angle is increased. Either weakness or underuse of the gluteals (the buttock muscles) will have the same net effect as tightness of the muscles that flex the hip joint. If the long muscles in the back of the spine, the prime movers, are tight or go into spasm (a condition of continuous contraction), it also increases the lumbo-sacral angle. The prime movers go into this state of prolonged spasm because there is inadequate stabilization of one or more vertebral joints. The attempt to stabilize the joint for any particular motion is carried out in the central nervous system far below the conscious level. If the individual were fully aware of what was happening, he might think: "I would like to bend my trunk 15° to the left front, but the stabilization at L4-5 is not adequate, therefore I will put two muscles of group L1-4 and three muscles of group R2-5 into heavier contraction. But as I do this I increase the shearing force at L4-5 further and cause more abnormal ligament stretch. This is now exciting pain fibers that are registering in the pain network. Shall I go ahead with awareness of pain or shall I give it its full due? Decisions!"

No, the process is without this anatomical observation. If so much awareness was inherent in every move, there would be little time for anything else. The higher executive, the mind, sets the broad policy—"I will bend"—and the various components strive to fulfill their function without bothering the planner. If they do not work well, all that is brought forth into the consciousness is: "There is pain and stiffness. The motion is poor. Will I pay attention to it or not?"

When any portion of the body is functioning well we are unaware of its existence. If we are conscious of a foot at every step, then something is wrong. Similarly, if there is an awareness of the back at every movement, something is amiss.

The person who seeks help for his back must certainly be aware of it. He has not been able to will it back into the almost forgotten section of his mind. As we shall see, the initial phase of helping the situation will be to increase the awareness of the back. This is done by improving the action and the interaction of the involved muscles. As a result of this there is most often an alteration in posture. The direction of this change is towards the reduction of the lumbo-sacral angle as a means of lessening the strain in the region, which will enable the stabilization system to move efficiently. In effect, it will provide for better action on the part of the prime movers.

The individual will be helped if in the final stage he can cary his load of daily activities without feeling that he has a back. The posture that enables him to do this will be assumed almost without thought, and will be natural without strain.

Of course, you cannot look at a person and say, "Your posture is all wrong—you are sure to develop back trouble!" because, though the posture is "bad" or inefficient, the demands on that back may not be large enough to reveal the weakness. But once a back in that category has been stressed sufficiently, the difficulty may require postural training to restore the former carefree state.

There are many people who have a marked lordosis—sometimes called "swayback"—in which the lumbo-sacral angle is markedly increased. In these people there is a built-in compensatory strengthening of the local muscle and ligament systems. But after an injury or under conditions where the system can no longer compensate, the return to normal back function may present additional difficulties.

Good posture for proper function does not mean, as might be thought, a stiff forced bearing in which the muscular effort causes a constant tenseness. It would be well to resurrect a most unused word—carriage. The word expresses posture in motion. A good carriage used to mean an appropriate erect bearing, which exerted a feeling of presence, proper esteem, or property. Although it projected this, we are more interested in its physical aspects —good muscular action. It is hoped that with the improvement in muscular control good carriage will come naturally.

6

Types of
Low Back Derangement

To THE RELATIVELY uninformed there is only "back trouble." The better informed knows of "back trouble" and a "disc," but for the physician with a wider observation, there are both qualitative and quantitative varieties of low back difficulties. There are backaches that occur with only minor trauma, with x-rays showing normal bone structure or congenital abnormalities. There are acute back conditions and chronic ones. The chronic ones can vary from a fairly constant state of discomfort during any activity or repeated attacks of extremely severe pain.

The low back derangement can exist in as many varieties as any other disease form. For example, measles, a disease that should produce a rash, may exist without a skin eruption. As the back condition can be present in different states, the treatment for one state may be different from that for another.

With the above in mind, let us see how some of these different varieties of low back derangement present themselves and how the mechanical basis so far presented will help to explain the differences. A starting point would be the history of the onset of these conditions.

The first example would be a sudden wrench. This

might occur in a vehicular accident, or result from a slip or fall, or even from walking down a staircase and misjudging the last step. The injury is usually the result of a sudden violent muscle contraction. The contraction might come as a direct result of the local trauma or may be the result of a sudden tensing to ward off the blow. It is possible that this tensing prior to the blow can cause more injury than the blow itself. Because of this (the reaction to the impending injury), there may be more than one level of injury to the spine. If the patient falls on his buttocks there may be an injury to the buttocks region, a injury direct to the sciatic nerve or by indirect force to the lower lumbar spine. In a great many cases the indirect injury is of far more consequence than the direct injury.

Examples of the pure indirect injuries are those produced by high tension electric shocks that activate the spinal muscles. Though the point of application of the electricity is nowhere near the back, the sudden violent contraction of the muscles can cause torn ligaments, fractures and dislocations in the spine.

Pain frequently occurs when an individual straightens up after having been in a cramped or awkward position for a while. The story of the occurrence of pain when activity (trunk motion) is resumed after a period of inactivity is also common. In a sense, the same thing occurs when an individual suddenly sneezes without warning, and starts the back pain. The related story of back pain after sudden episodes of vomiting or coughing is also common.

Although, at first glance, for many of these a pre-existing ligamentous weakness or bone abnormality might seem to be the cause, another explanation is possible. For some reason, the muscles involved did not act together in a proper pattern. The pattern for muscular interaction had "gone to sleep"—did not respond smoothly on sudden demand. The prime movers started a forceful contraction before the stabilization muscles were ready and pulled the joint apart. Or the stabilization muscles clamped down too soon and too hard and momentarily froze the joint, which caused an intolerable strain within the prime movers. The effect of the abnormal stress to the joint structure or connected musculature can result in any degree of strain or even a tear.

A direct trauma to the back, such as would result from falling on the edge of a stair or railing, may also be the cause of the difficulty. Or the force may be in the axis of the spine, as in a fall from a height. A transverse blow to the back can cause a fracture of bone at any level depending on the impact region. The fall from a height is most apt to cause a fracture at the point where the movable lumbar spine meets the relatively fixed thoracic spine or the sacrum. The major injury, then, occurs either at the upper or lower end of the lumbar spine. But, as noted previously, besides the direct injury there can be an indirect injury because of the sudden uncontrollable reflex contraction of the abdominal, trunk and spine muscles.

It is a good time to point out that not all bodily reactions (involuntary and voluntary) to an injury or an impending injury are beneficial to the individual. Many of the varieties of defensive reaction to a disturbance may harm the person if they are too strong or continued too long. An allergic response is such a reaction.

The bodily damage produced by a trauma is very often dependent on the individual. When a baby just learning to walk falls, very little is hurt. He falls softly, rolling limply with the blow. But, as the child gets older, a learned fear reaction sets in. This may be influenced by parental reaction to the thought of an injury. When the child starts to fall now, fear makes him stiffen up and the rigidity of his body causes injury. As part of this, the timing of bodily reactions will have a strong influence. The classic illustration puts three men in a darkened room. The men are the same height, and the same weight, but have different emotional reactions. Across the width of the room is strung an unseen wire just high enough to trip them. The men walk across the room in a natural fashion. Though the men are similar in many ways, when they trip, different things happen. One is uninjured, one breaks a wrist, and the last one breaks an ankle. The explanation has to do with the time of onset of the fear or stiffening reaction. The individual who did not develop it in time fell softly. The one who developed it quickly injured his ankle. The one who developed it more slowly stiffened as he threw out his hand to break the fall and injured the wrist. The injury then was not determined by the situation or the defensive reaction. It was related to the time at which the reaction occurred after the initial warning. In a general way, though this timing is not under direct control, it can be modified by training, as in the case of an acrobat who has learned how to fall, or a fighter who has learned to roll with the punch. The time it takes to learn and the completeness of the learning is not the same for all.

We can now look at the effects of trauma on the vertebral body and its attachments. A force can cause a strained muscle or ligament; the structure is pulled beyond its normal tolerance. There is some immediate back pain. If the strain is very mild not much else happens. If the strain is more severe, an inflammatory fluid collects in the tissues. The fluid is derived from the blood and resembles blood without the cells. As the fluid collects it distends the tissues and puts pressure on the nerve endings, which is felt as pain. If it collects in the muscles, the muscles feel stiff. The reaction can build up to give delayed pain and stiffness. The patient may feel more pain and stiffness the next day. An example of this type of delayed reaction occurs when an out-of-practice individual rows a boat for a few hours. The next day he may have such sore abdominal muscles as to give rise to speculation that he has peritonitis.

In a sprain, the trauma is severe enough to have caused a tear in a ligament or muscle. It may not go all the way across. It may involve only the internal fibers of the structure without tearing the outside covering layer. If a telephone cable containing many strands of wire is hit with a soft heavy hammer it is possible to sever some of the wires inside the cable without breaking the outer insulating cover. In a sprain, the reaction in the tissues is more immediate. Fluid and even whole blood from torn blood vessels may pour out into the tissues. The patient feels severe pain immediately which then merges into any delayed reaction.

At times the force is so directed that a ligament or tendon will not tear in its course but pull out of the bone, or more usually pull out a piece of bone. This is called a sprain fracture or an avulsion fracture. The fact that there is a fracture is not as important as the loss in continuity of the ligament. It has the same overall effect as a torn ligament.

A contusion occurs at the point where the blow is struck. How much damage is done will depend on many factors—the force of the blow, the area of impact and the resistance of the tissues. A contusion of any significance will cause bleeding into the tissues which subsequently takes on different coloration because of the breakdown of the blood pigments. The significance of the injury does not depend on the size and color of the pigmented area but on the bruising of the underlying structures.

All the above tissue injuries can happen to any part of the body—to an ankle, arm, or wrist—and it is now important to see what peculiarities occur in the back that make its injuries a source of so much difficulty.

The first most obvious feature is that the injured tissues in the back are deeper, more difficult to feel by the examiner, more difficult to localize by the patient. There is less ability to accurately localize a source of pain in the back than in other portions of the body. If two sharp points are placed one-eighth inch apart on the tongue, there will be recognition of the fact that there are two points. If the same two points are placed on the skin of the back, they will feel like one point. This same ability or inability to distinguish closely exists beneath the surface. The patient cannot tell if his fourth or second lumbar vertebra is the source of his pain. All he knows is that there is back pain.

If the injury has caused a strain there will be regional, diffuse low back pain. It may be on one or both sides, depending on the structures involved. The motion disturbance in the back will not be great, and the condition will gradually resolve on almost any kind of treatment—provided the method is not too abusive—or none.

The sprain is perhaps the most important of low back injuries. If the sprain involves the large muscles or liga-

Figure 19a. A normal relationship; 10—sacrum; 11—ilium; 9—fulcrum stabilizing system (small muscles and ligaments); 12—prime movers (the large muscles).

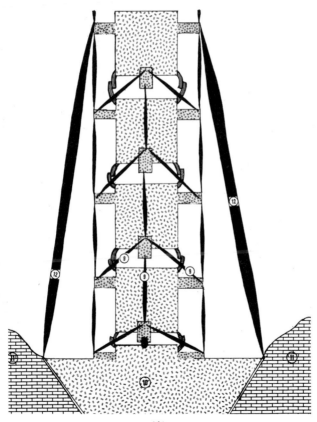

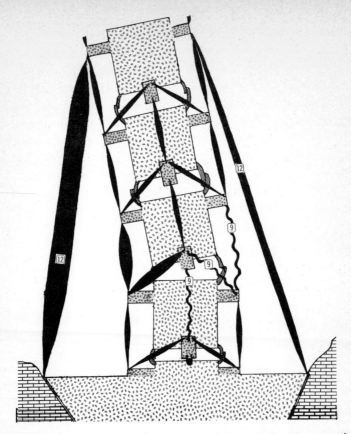

Figure 19b. Acute back derangement (sciatic skoliosis); note tilt. 9—faulty stabilizing system; 12—long muscles in spasm in an attempt to stabilize the spine.

ments of the spine system, the pain may be rather widespread, and the discomfort and stiffness on motion will be more persistent. It will require more active treatment than the strain and may leave behind it a residue of pain and stiffness with heavy back stress. If the sprain is severe and involves the small muscles or ligaments of the fulcrum establishment system (the vertebral joint stabilization system) described previously, then more serious difficulties will be encountered. The prime movers attempt by over-contraction to stabilize the defective hinge—the point at which motion should occur. The attempt to have the joint act as a pivot for motion or a stabilizer to maintain a posture will cause the forceful, though sometimes futile, over-contraction of the muscles. But the direction of their action is not in the proper line to stabilize the joint, and the more they pull, the more they can move the joint surfaces away from their position of stability. The resulting instability may send the signals for even more unwanted contraction. Because of the forceful contraction of the prime movers which can be greater on one side, the entire trunk may list or shift to one side. This tilt of the trunk is called a scoliosis. When it is accompanied by pain it is generally called an acute sciatic scoliosis. This is only a descriptive term used to state the position or appearance of the condition and does not tell exactly where the injured tissues are. (Figure 19.)

Frequently the pain is concentrated over the left or right lower portion of the back at the upper portion of the pelvis, or, more accurately, where the sacrum joins the pelvis. This is the region of the sacro-iliac joints and, as noted previously, the diagnosis of sacro-iliac sprain at one time was considered fitting and proper for the condition. But it is also a major point of attachment of the important prime mover muscle. It is now felt that the pain at this point is caused by the forceful contraction of the muscle and the resulting heavy pull at its attachment point.

If the back force is so directed as to also (or only) cause a severe sprain of the ligament that surrounds the disc, the disc substance will be forced out. The rupture of this ligament can happen after one severe trauma. It can also occur after a relatively minor trauma (a sneeze or cough or a bend) if the structural properties of the ligament have been damaged by other minor trauma or repeated unnatural stresses. At this point, a word about common usage. Although the term in general use; "slipped disc," is picturesque, it is not very accurate. The disc, normally composed of a firm jellylike substance, cannot slip out of place like a poker chip; it oozes out. The word "slipped" is a carry-over from the recent past when back troubles were supposed to result from a sacro-iliac joint that slipped out of place.

When the disc substance forces its way out at the side where the nerve roots (Figure 16, page 37) emerge, there will usually be pain in the region that the nerve root supplies. The back pain may be relatively minor and most often will gradually decrease. Accompanying the initial back pain there will also usually be spasm of the back muscles in an involuntary attempt to stabilize and splint that vertebral segment that is causing the nerve root irritation.

The pain in the lower extremity depends on how hard the nerve root (or roots) is compressed by the disc substance. The location of the pain depends on which root is affected. If the root is one that supplies a portion of the leg there will be pain that seems to originate in the leg. The leg muscles that are controlled by that nerve root may be affected, and can be weakened to the point of paralysis. Often, before the weakness can be noted, the deep tendon reflex will be decreased. If the tendon the deep tendon reflex will be decreased.

If sufficient pressure is made the reflex may be completely absent. The pressure on the nerve can cause decreased sensation in the area of skin supplied by the nerve. There may be both pain, of several varieties, and numbness in the same area of the skin.

Up to now the descriptions have been concerned with the effects of trauma on relatively normal backs. But not all backs (or spines and their muscular and ligament attachments) fall into this group. A spine may be abnormal and the bone elements of this abnormality can be seen on an x-ray. If there is a soft tissue abnormality, which may make for weakness, it will not be revealed by ordinary x-ray examination, unless there is a bone abnormality associated with it. Some of the abnormalities are directly associated with the inability of the back to stand up under any unusual stress. The discussion of the most common types of bone abnormality, and their meaning, will be found in Chapter 7.

7

Repair Ability

IN THE PREVIOUS discussion the injury effects have seemed to go in an unhappy downhill course. A trauma known or unknown has led stepwise to a herniated intervertebral disc. But life and the body do not always work against us. The process can stop anywhere along the line. It must be evident that statistically this is so, as almost everyone has had back trauma or unusual stress at some time in their life, but the whole population does not walk around with a crippled back.

The course may be stopped if the effects of the trauma heal, if the back is not stressed again beyond its limits, if the injury effects can be circumvented or if some physical compensation can be made.

The healing process should be considered first. It has been noted that, in a strain, there is no loss of structural strength. The damage to the tissues gives rise to a mild inflammatory process in which fluid accumulates in and between the tissues. Gradually the fluid is absorbed; its absorption rate can usually be helped by mild heat, gentle motion and medication. Measures that tend to increase the blood supply to the involved region all help. When the inflammatory fluid is absorbed or dissipated, the tissues are practically as good as new. The back has the physical ability to be stressed again, as hard as it was before. The injury does not make it especially vulnerable to another injury. (Except if the individual is too careful and over-reacts to an impending injury.)

In a sprain there is a structural tear within the tissue. A ligament, tendon or muscle is torn. Or a tendon or ligament may tear away from its boney attachment. Most often the tear is incomplete; it occurs within the substance of the structure involved. The tears do not remain in the torn state. Given half a chance, i.e., not being over-stressed within the healing period, a repair will be made with fibrous tissue, the type of tissue of which scars are made. The tendon or ligament contains elastic tissue. Elastic tissue has give; it can absorb a great deal of stress without tearing. The fibrous tissue does not have the same amount of give, but still it is a repair and can take a reasonable load. The once-torn, inadequate ligament or tendon can again be used. The tear in the muscle also heals with a fibrous scar. Naturally the scar does not have the same ability to contract as does the muscle but it can maintain a continuity—the line of pull. Given enough time and nourishment, the scar will contract down to the point where it is indistinguishable from the original tissue. It is a familiar phenomenon that a deep cut on the skin will gradually contract down. A difficulty with tendons and ligaments more than with muscle, is the fact that they do not have a rich blood supply. As a result, their rate of change is not rapid. The final phase of healing may be quite slow.

The next injury is the extruded disc. As the disc substance is like a rubbery thickened jelly, it tends to stay together. It just does not flow easily out of harm's way. Once a rent has occurred in the surrounding ligament and the disc substance comes out, the pressure in the disc space keeps the substance from going back easily. The pressure is maintained by the weight of the body and also by the action of the spinal musculature. In most cases the weakness of the retaining ring for the disc has been the result of abnormal stabilization of the two vertebrae involved. The continuation of the abnormal stabilization tends to cause the increase in pressure within the disc space. Many neurosurgeons feel that a weakness in the disc retaining wall that permits it to bulge like a "bubble" in an automobile tire, has less of a chance of self-repair than does a full extrusion of disc substance. The extruded disc substance may return if the disc space pressure can be lowered. This is done by rest and relieving muscle spasm. The portion of disc substances can pinch off and drop down to the bottom of the dural sac where it is of little consequence. (The dural sac is the membrane that forms a bag containing the cushioning fluid that surrounds the central nervous system.)

If the disc substance pushes out in such a fashion as to make pressure on a nerve root, two effects occur. The first is the result of direct pressure. The second is the inflammatory response within the nerve root as a result of the bruising that the disc causes. It might be wondered how a relatively soft substance like a disc can cause damage to a nerve trunk which is actually firmer. It does this by interfering with the blood supply within the nerve root; it requires very little external pressure to impede the blood flow. The pressure also interferes with the flow of cell fluids in the nerve cell portion that forms the root.

In many cases the direct pressure of the disc material is not as important as the inflammatory reaction it causes. The disc substance may have gone its way (dropped off or gone back into place), but the inflamed swollen nerve root may still cause trouble. It can cause pain and neurological warning signs even though whatever started the reaction is no longer operative. When the inflammatory reaction subsides, the patient's complaints will also fade away. If the pressure on the nerve root has been considerable and the inflammatory response has been large for a long period of time, scars may be produced. The scars may be within the nerve root or between the root and its surroundings. These are what are familiarly called adhesions. Not all discs extrude out in such a fashion as to put pressure on a nerve root. Those that do not exert pressure on a root will not signal their presence by pain in the extremity. Only the backache will be present.

The tear in the annulus fibrosis, the surrounding ligament of the disc, undergoes changes with time. It can heal with the formation of a scar. If the scar is weak and there is still a large amount of disc substance or if the force on the disc set up continues to be abnormal, then another herniation or outward pouching of the disc substance can happen.

In most cases, if the patient has had a severe attack (often meaning a large outpouring of disc material), it is rare to have a second severe attack at the same level. Disc substance is not reformed in any appreciable amount and so another massive outpouring would not be probable. An attack at one level (for example, L5-S1) does not give immunity for an attack at another level (for example, L4-5).

If a great many people over thirty-five are x-rayed it will be found that many will have a narrowed interspace (meaning loss of disc substance) most frequently at L5-S1, next most frequently at L4-5. (In the neck, in the cervical spine, C5-6 narrowing is most frequent.) In the group that shows the lumbar interspace narrowing there may be some who have a history of back difficulties and some with a history of radiating pain down the extremity, but also some who have no history of any major back difficulty. The last group is most interesting. It might be said that the individuals in this group were insensitive to pain. A little investigation will show that this could not have been the reason. It is most probable that the individuals in this group have had a long-standing low back derangement. The stress of their activities has caused small outpourings of disc substance which did not press on a nerve root. The few episodes of low back discomfort can be attributed to a chill from an air conditioner, too much walking the day before on a shopping trip or sitting in a cramped position on the bus. It is also possible that, with age and the continued stress of abnormal motion—because of faulty intervertebral stabilization—the disc substance degenerated and shrunk. The degeneration of animal substances through too much motion can be seen in an example drawn from the kitchen. If cream is beaten too much, the whipped cream will turn into butter. This occurs because the milk proteins become denatured and shrink to an insoluble substance that can no longer hold the "whipped" state.

After looking through the pile of x-rays it will be discovered that many more people have back trouble than have been aware of it. It will also be obvious that it requires experience and skill to relate the patients' complaints and clinical findings to the x-ray findings.

8

The Role of the Physician

THE GENERAL DESCRIPTION of the anatomical elements in a low back derangement have now been presented. The question must now arise—what is the role of the physician in the treatment of the condition? His first major role is the determination of whether the condition that the patient presents is a back derangement and not some other condition that requires a completely different form of treatment. If, for example, the patient's back pain is caused by a kidney abscess, or inflammation in an abnormally situated appendix, then treatment with a diathermy apparatus is hardly helpful. So the first element is diagnosis as to location.

His next important function is to estimate the amount of the disease that is present. He must decide if the descriptions and the reactions of the patient fall into a normal range: if the patient is one in whom a small amount of pain causes major complaints and severe disability, or if the patient is one who tries to ignore physical discomfort. By the time the patient seeks help the condition has progressed to the extent that simple measures will not do. And, of course, there is the group to whom the disability projected from a back condition is such an important part of existence that any attempt to help is rejected either openly or in a disguised fashion. The last group looks upon every little pain or ache as an indicator of the most serious form of disease. Throughout their narrative there is the fear that their body will do them in. These groups are mentioned because the total personality factor is important in estimating the value of the history given by the patient.

From the patient's history the physician finds out if the attack is acute or only one of a series of attacks. The precipitating feature of the attack can be brought out; i.e., did it come on after a sneeze, or was there a fall on a stairs, or did it happen when the patient was thrown about in a car accident or fell from a tilting chair. It is important to know if the difficulty is only back pain or if there is radiation into the leg, and does the pain persist at rest. If the leg pain is severe now, did it start at once or was the back pain the first feature. And is it a matter of sharp pain or mostly a matter of dull ache. All these points are important for the final estimate of the condition.

The next point is the physical examination. The observation of the way in which the patient moves or stands is part of the examination. The patient can have a tilted trunk because of muscle spasm. Or, the trunk may be tilted because one leg is shorter. The constant tilt imposed by unequal leg length may cause a continuing strain on the back. Though the ligaments and muscles can withstand the strain for a long time, they may show an increasing reaction to it and so produce evidence of their distress. Or an injury may cause some damage which does not heal properly because of the element of constant strain.

The movements of the spine can reveal a great deal about its state. Severe muscle spasm may prevent all motion or may permit it in only one direction. The physician can feel for tenderness. He can note if it is present in the spine or in the muscles alongside of it. It is also possible for the pain to arise from pelvic structures, either ligaments or the sciatic nerve. Often the pain arising from the pelvic structure can closely mimic that coming from the spine. And it is only by careful examination, external and internal, that the distinction can be made.

Among other conditions that can cause more strain than the normal back can tolerate is an arthritic condition of the hips. The presence of limited hip motion can impose added strain on the vertebral joints in maintaining the upright posture. Motion of the hips to the pelvis is limited. The rotary and flexion movements and the displacements that are the result of alternate foot weight bearing in walking and which are normally absorbed in the pelvis and hip joint must now be passed on to the spine. This added stress over the years may ultimately be more than the spinal joints can tolerate.

After having observed the musculo-skeletal effects of the back disturbance, an evaluation of possible neurological effects must be checked. This is done by noting the strength of the key muscles and noting if there are any areas of disturbed sensation. The amount and duration of nerve compression will determine how these functions are affected. If the nerve pressure has been severe for a length of time, atrophy or wasting of the related tissues will also have occurred. The reflexes which are brought forth by a sharp tap on a tendon give information by the rapidity and strength of response.

It takes a certain amount of experience to appreciate these reactions and to know when there is a significant departure from the normal. Often it is difficult for the average lay person to appreciate the fact that many of the things that are observed for the making of a diagnosis are quite subtle. Further, it is just not one thing alone—a spot of tenderness, a reflex or a movement—that furnishes a working diagnosis. The significant factors have to be picked and then properly combined if the findings are to have meaning.

A proper examination should also include x-ray studies. The x-rays can reveal many factors that have importance for the diagnosis. Although the ordinary x-rays will show only bone detail, soft tissue abnormalities can be projected into the image through proper interpretation.

NORMAL

In a normal x-ray, there should be the normal number of boney parts. The bone should have a proper density, which means that it has the right mineral content. The curve of the lumbar spine as seen in a side projection (lateral view) should resemble the curve illustrated in Figure 3, page 18. A straightening of the curve is indicative of spasm of the long muscles of the back, either as a direct response to injury, an attempt to splint a painful joint, or a try to stabilize a joint whose stabilization apparatus is faulty.

NARROWED INTERSPACE

A narrowed interspace is indicative of a loss in intervertebral disc volume which can come about through degeneration of disc substance followed by shrinkage or by loss of disc substance either through a rent in the surrounding ligament or into the bone substance on either side. A great many people over thirty-five have a decrease in one or more intervertebral spaces, usually L5-S1 or L4-L5. It is at this level that most stress has been applied to the spinal column. The stress of one episode or repeated episodes has caused inadequacy of the stabilization system which results in the "wearing out" of the surrounding ligament—annulus fibrosus. Careful examination of the narrowing can often furnish information on whether the narrowing is new or old. An old narrowing has changes at the attachment of the ligaments and in the related joints. The changes are little spikes of bone and local increases in bone density (increased mineral content). The new disc space narrowing shows none of these reactive changes. The determination of whether the

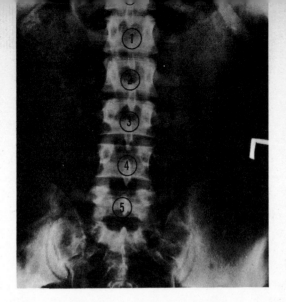

Figure 20a. Normal spine. X-ray front to back, showing the five lumbar vertebrae.

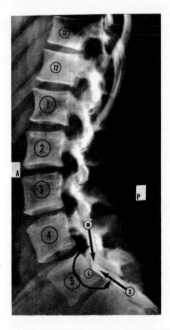

Figure 20b. Normal spine, side view, showing the five lumbar vertebrae. A—front; P—back; W—direction of weight force; S—direction of supporting force; L—angle at lumbo-sacral junction, which shows the shearing force.

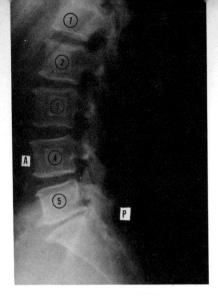

Figure 21. Narrowed interspace, side view. A—front; P—back. The narrowed interspace is between the fifth lumbar vertebrae (5) and the sacrum; narrowing to a much lesser degree is present between the fourth lumbar (4) and the fifth lumbar (5).

narrowing is new or old may play a significant role. If the disc space narrowing is old, it may have less meaning with relation to the episode under investigation.

ARTHRITIC CHANGES

The spine is subject to arthritic changes. There are many types of arthritis ranging from a direct infectious arthritis which can be caused by a variety of micro-organisms from the tubercle bacillus to other forms that are still not identified.

The arthritis that is most often encountered is hypertrophic arthritis. Other names have been applied to this —i.e., senescent arthritis and degenerative arthritis—but these are unhappy terms to use. The favored term is osteoarthritis. The term is derived from bone spurs and the increases in bone density at points of strain. For simplicity's sake and ease of discussion, the arthritis is often presumed to be the cause of the back pain and disability. Actually it is not a cause but really an effect.

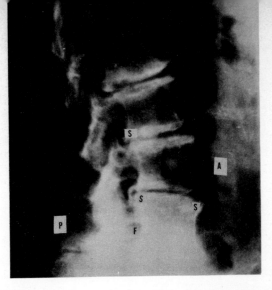

Figure 22. Osteoarthritis in lumbar spine, side view. Note irregular dense bone laid down at stressed regions. A—front; P—back; S—arthritic spurs which encroach on foramen (nerve passageway) (F) in backward direction. Note also the narrowed interspaces between the vertebral bodies, which means that the disc has degenerated.

It is caused by the faulty action of the muscles and ligaments that act on the bones. The hypertrophic bone changes are the tissue responses in the individual to the stresses applied to the region. In the young individuals such tissue strains are easily dissipated and repaired well. But with advancing age (and in some individuals the tendency is greater) the localized strains cause the changes. The basic aim of treatment at present for this type of arthritis is not aimed directly at the arthritis. Because in actuality the arthritic changes are just evidence that prior to the time of observation the joints and ligament attachments were strained beyond their tolerance. The aim of treatment is to improve muscle function and relieve abnormal ligament and joint strain. This will minimize further arthritic formation. (Figure 22.)

The other forms of arthritis are not specifically related to the problem of low back derangement except that they have to be excluded as a basis of the difficulty, in individual cases, before instituting treatment.

FRACTURES

Fractures can occur in various portions of the vertebrae. Again, only the most common one will be considered. The other types, though very important to the
individual, cannot be dealt with here. This also applies
to dislocations between the vertebrae. As in a skull fracture, it is not the bone injury that is of major importance,
but the injury to the contained nerve tissue.

The most common injury encountered is the compression fracture of the vertebral body. The body is compressed, the greatest compression occurring in front. Early
in this century, heroic measures were undertaken to relieve the compression. Since World War II it has become
increasingly evident that the unseen injury in the soft
tissues was a lot more important than the fracture seen
in the x-ray. It can be said that this concept did much
to enliven and give force to the whole field of rehabilitation. Medical efforts at present are directed more towards

Figure 23.   Fracture.

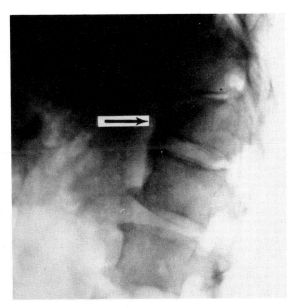

the rehabilitation of the soft tissues—muscles, ligaments and tendons—rather than doing anything specific about the fracture.

It must be realized that when a patient sustains a fracture the soft-tissue stressing just before the bone crushes can give rise to a low back derangement at that level. A great percentage of the fractures occur in the upper lumbar spine, L1, L2, L3. However, that region may not be the only one stressed before the bone breaks. It is possible, and it frequently happens, that the soft tissues of the L5-S1 or L4-5 level are also injured. (Figure 23.)

As a final note on fractures, it has been frequently observed that a compressed vertebrae can be found on an x-ray. A careful questioning of the patient will often fail to disclose a history of either a serious accident or prolonged disability. Again, it must be concluded that since the soft tissue injuries were not severe, the patient was not cognizant of the other effect (bone injury) of the trauma.

CONGENITAL EFFECTS

There are several congenital abnormalities of the spine. Often these abnormalities mean little, but at times the pressure of some of them seem to make the back more vulnerable to stress. The common forms are:

1. *Numerical alteration:* In this there may be either more (6) or less (4) lumbar vertebrae. Since five is the normal number, it would seem likely that the abnormal number makes for a setup that can be more vulnerable to the stress occuring in a normally active life. If the remark seems to be somewhat hedging, it is no accident. There is a fair amount of uncertainty on this point because of lack of adequate surveys as to the potentialities of this abnormality.

2. *Spina Bifida Occulta:* This unwieldy diagnosis refers to a failure of the boney elements to fuse over the top

(or back) of the spinal canal. At one time this finding was blamed for some other conditions—for example, bed-wetting. Now it is felt to be relatively unimportant with regard to causing or setting the stage for back instability.

3. *Spondylolisthesis:* This is caused by a pedicle defect. The pedicle is the little bridge of bone between the joints and the body of the vertebrae. In time the vertebral body will usually slip forward. The upper vertebrae may also be carried forward, or one vertebral body can go forward alone. There is reasonable doubt whether the condition is always of congenital origin. There are reported cases in which the condition has been caused by force which resulted in fractures through the pedicles which did not heal. The symptoms can range from an ordinary backache to nerve root compression because of the altered relationship of the bones. Though the condition can make its presence felt in adolescence, most frequently the individual is unaware of it until past thirty. An injury may cause some damage which permits the vertebrae to go from the pre-slip stage to the slipped stage. Or this may happen gradually with a slow

Figure 24. Spondyolisthesis. A—front; P—back. Note the break in continuity of the black line which traces the posterior (back) border of the vertebral bodies. This is caused by the forward slip of 4 in relation to 5.

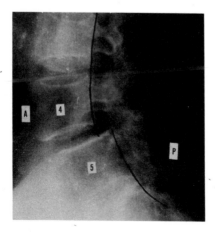

buildup of symptoms. When the slippage is such that there is nerve root pressure, treatment to relieve the pressure should be started without delay. (Figure 24.)

A final word on diagnosis. There are conditions that can resemble, from the history, and even from the findings from the x-rays, varieties of low back derangement with or without radiating pain. Even the special tests commonly employed may not provide a good answer. In such a case it may take a great deal of skill and imagination to arrive at a useful diagnosis.

SPECIAL TESTS

1. *Lumbar Puncture*. This consists of inserting a needle into the spinal canal to determine the pressure of the spinal fluid and withdraw a sample for analysis. Where there is strong indication of a herniated disc, the lumbar puncture is usually done as part of a myelogram (see below). By itself it is an important part of the neurological examination.

2. *Myelogram*. This consists of injecting a substance into the spinal canal to outline any protrusions into the canal. The substance injected is of greater density than the soft tissue of the canal and shows up on the x-ray screen, thus revealing any irregularities. The injected material is usually withdrawn after this procedure.

3. *Discogram*. In certain institutions this is a popular procedure. It consists of injecting a chemical into the disc substance which will make it (the disc) visible on the x-ray screen.

4. *Electrodiagnostic Study*. This procedure measures the conduction and strength of the electrical impulses in nerves and the structures they serve. It has proven to be of great value and will undoubtedly become an even more useful tool in the future.

TREATMENT

The endeavor, to this point, has been to show that low back difficulty can exist in more than one form. For practical purposes these forms can be listed as:

1. Acute: a) without radiation
            b) with radiation
2. Recurrent
3. Chronic

ACUTE FORM WITHOUT RADIATING PAIN

In this there is back pain, stiffness and, at times, a tilt or shift of the trunk. The pain is caused not only by the local inflammation in the muscles, ligament and joint capsule but also by muscle spasm. The muscle spasm is an effort of part of the body's defense system to stop motion at a painful region. If the particular segment cannot be stabilized because the small muscle ligament system or joint system is inadequate, the long muscles contract in an effort to stabilize the system. The local inadequacy is either a direct result of the injury or the inflammatory response evoked by the effects of the injury.

The muscle spasm, which is defensive, may, if continued too long, be detrimental or prevent the easy resolution of the back difficulty. The forceful muscle spasm exerts a pull in a direction that is not proper to stabilize the joint and so can cause further abnormal stress on the joint. This may in turn cause further inflammation. It is a vicious circle which aggravates itself, making the circle tighter and more durable.

There are various ways to break this circle. Sometimes, if the trouble is mild, just rest will do it. If the inflammatory element is most important, an anti-inflammatory agent will do it. If the muscle spasm is the most prominent feature, attacking that element may be enough. Often both the spasm and the inflammation may have to be dealt with together to effectively open the circle. There are both medical and physical measures to ac-

71

complish this and many of these measures work simultaneously on both inflammation and spasm. An example is gentle heat which allays an inflammatory response and also relaxes muscles.

Medical anti-inflammatory measures consist of medications that can range from Aspirin through the Cortisone products. In addition, there are some synthetic anti-inflammatory chemicals and some enzyme products derived from both animal and plant sources. Many physicians prefer to inject anti-inflammatory medication directly into a suspected region. This produces a high concentration at the region of involvement. To obtain such a high concentration by taking the medicine by mouth would lead to an almost equally high concentration in other tissues. This might cause unwelcome side effects. Local injection of procaine (T. M.—Novocaine) into the back may be one of the measures that has an overlapping effect; it not only causes local muscle paralysis to relieve spasm but may also have a mild anti-inflammatory action.

Two other forms of physical energy can be used, diathermy and ultrasonic radiation. When diathermy is used, very short length radio waves are passed through the tissues. As the waves have such short wave length it is possible to control their direction. The function of diathermy is to cause a warming of the deep tissues. It is widely believed that the deep heat produced is the only factor of importance; the radio waves themselves have no specific properties.

In ultrasonic radiation, very high frequency sound waves are applied to the tissue. For a long time there have been heated discussions in medical circles on whether the ultrasonic vibrations had any other effect in addition to the deep heat it produced. In any case, the deep heat does function as a useful agent.

The muscle-relaxing medications are numerous. For the most part they are taken by mouth, though some can be taken intravenously—under careful medical supervision, of course. To date, most of these, despite manufacturers' claims, have been short of miraculous in effect, since the dose would produce effective relief of spasm verges closely on the dose that would cause uncomfortable side effects.

A method of relieving muscle spasm (or perhaps relieving inflammation) is the application of sudden temperature changes to the skin. Spraying the skin over the affected regions with a highly volatile liquid such as ethyl chloride causes a pronounced local cooling. This is not frequently used, however, since its effectiveness is limited to very mild cases.

Massage, of the non-abusive type, also has value. There are devotees of the various forms of massage, from easy skin stroking to a subtle form of Karate with alternate chopping with both sides of the hand. But it has always seemed to be effective in only the milder cases. For some, the personal contact is a more satisfying experience, and so there is an added fringe benefit to induce relaxation of taut muscle groups.

Among the most popular methods in use to cut down on muscle spasm are the manipulative methods. In these one portion of the body is made to move with relation to the other. Some manipulative procedures aim to have a vertebra move against other vertebrae by direct pressure application over the vertebra.

A word of caution is in order at this point. If the patient has evidence of nerve root irritation, as indicated by signs and symptoms in a leg, abrupt, forceful manipulation may aggravate or produce further nerve root pressure.

In general, manipulative treatment may be divided into two general types—traction or a relatively slow gradual pulling, mostly in one direction, and a manual forceful twisting, bending and/or stretching, usually done in a rapid fashion.

73

TRACTION

There are several forms of traction. Most commonly used today is the pelvic belt which is pulled down by means of weights attached to cords which are then attached to either side of the pelvic belt. Some years ago the point of attachment of the traction force to the legs was more popular but, of late, the pelvic traction has been considered more useful. Opinions as to the application of force are not uniform. Some physicians have obtained good results with a gentle steady force while others feel brief periods of very strong traction is of greater value. To be diplomatic, it is best said that both have been helpful in reducing spasm, but that deriving benefit from one form does not rule out the possibility that another form will work too.

MANUAL MANIPULATION

If this form of exerting force is analyzed it will be seen that its action is very similar to an intermittent forceful traction with the addition of twisting and bending forces. Various maneuvers are done to accomplish this—either slowly or with a rapid jerking motion. Sometimes an audible snap is heard to everybody's satisfaction, and then someone says, "There, it's in!" which causes great relief all around—if "it" stays in. The nature of the snap is an interesting point for speculation. Very few really believe that the snap is caused by the sudden return of the disc to its rightful place, but it is an easy explanation which does not usually lead to further questions, so it satisfies without too much work. The two most accepted theories are (1) that the noise is produced by fibrous tissue or tight muscle slipping over a boney prominence, or (2) that it is the reduction of a subluxation. The slipping of a fibrous band is known to occur around other joints such as the hip.

Figure 25 shows congruous motions in a hypothetical

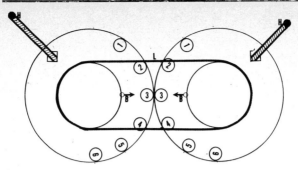

Figure 25a. Normal relationship in a joint. When hand H is moved, rotation of one wheel surface will cause the other to rotate and similar points will meet up. Force B, exerted by binding structure L, tends to maintain the alignment.

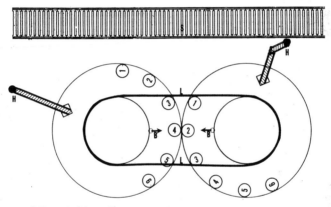

Figure 25b. Subluxed joint. Similar points no longer meet up. The binding force B tends to maintain the malalignment. Motion of the handles are restricted because of this; while one still has a distance to travel, the other has abutted against the stop S.

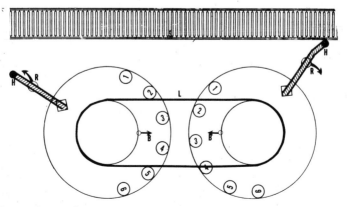

Figure 25c. The joint can be reduced back to normal by a new force R applied to the handles, which is sufficient to overcome binding force B.

joint. In the congruous motion the proper points always meet up. By shifting the pressure the joint bearing surfaces are altered; in effect, the relationships of the pivot points are changed. When this happens the motions are altered. Point 1 will meet up with point 3. An "internal subluxation" is produced. In this situation it will be seen that now the permitted range of motion of both halves of the joint is markedly limited—much less than the excursion for the marker arms (range of joint motion).

The subluxation tends to be maintained by the tension of the "ligaments" around the joint. Now the joint can be reduced by traction outward, whereupon it is "snatched" back into place by ligaments. The joint reduces with an audible snap. "There, it's in!" It is interesting that, in a model based on this, when the joint is markedly subluxed, traction must be instituted to disengage the joint surfaces before a reduction can be accomplished.

Another theory to explain the benefits derived from traction holds that the gradual pull relieves the spasm through a decrease in the excitability of muscle fibers.

There are many methods of application of the manipulative treatment. While some physicians feel that it is not a useful measure, others have demonstrated that it can produce relief in some patients. Most are agreed that it is not of itself curative, and that it cannot solve the problem of either preventing recurring acute attacks or setting to right a serious chronic low back derangement.

When the acute attack is accompanied by pain and radiation into the lower extremity the treatment should be more closely tied to the diagnosis. It is important to know early in the treatment if the pain is caused by pressure on a nerve root. The course of the patient under treatment should be watched to see if the signs and symptoms of nerve root pressure are subsiding or increasing. If they increase it can indicate that a surgical release must be considered.

In the patient with leg pain, care should be taken to avoid rapid forceful manipulation. Although this sign may simply indicate an inflamed nerve rather than direct disc substance pressure, it is better to avoid additional force, which might cause further pressure effects.

In the case of an inflamed nerve root, the aim of the treatment is rest for the injured part in order to prevent the nerve root from rubbing against the extruded disc substance or simply to avoid movement of inflamed tissue. And here is an advantage of traction: It forces the patient to rest under the most favorable circumstances. No practical way has been found to temporarily rest the spine without resting the whole body.

In most cases the severity or mildness of the initial attack of the back trouble does not give a good indication of what lies ahead. There are many people whose first mild attack is only the faintest prelude to a long series of attacks of ever-increasing severity. There are others who have a severe attack at first and do not have another for the next twenty years. More than one factor will determine the path taken. The damaged structures (usually not bones) may repair poorly or inadequately for the load imposed on them. Or the compensatory mechanism called into play may not be strong enough to make good for a long period or to override the damage. It may fail when the stress is too great.

There are two general routes that are taken when a low back derangement becomes chronic. One is recurring attacks with comparatively free normal intervals between the attacks. The other is a persistent low back pain, aggravated by any slight additional stress. Of course it is possible to have a great deal of overlapping of these two types.

Recurrent back aches can be precipitated by all varieties of stress, ranging from that caused by stepping off a curb in an awkward manner, sitting too long in a poorly designed seat, or even a violent sneeze. When the chronic back pain is constant, even when at rest in a good position, then it must be determined whether there is a source of the pain other than the derangement.

When the patient suffers a first not-too-severe attack which subsides well under treatment, then there does not seem to be much sense in undertaking a whole program of treatment. But if the attack is very severe or if it is one of a long series, then thought must be given to the rehabilition of the damaged back.

9

Chronic Low Back Derangement

To UNDERSTAND THE treatment for the persistent low back derangement it is necessary to take note of certain details. The first is that muscles which are used are stronger than those that are not used. Further, the structures associated with the muscles—the tendons, ligaments and bone—also become stronger through proper muscular action. When any of these structures are damaged, gradual use will be necessary to further the last stage of healing. In a chronic low back derangement a torn structure may not have been repaired properly. The repair by fibrous tissue (the scar) may not have the right "give" under a sudden load. The repair may be responsible for shortening or the scar may adhere to nearby muscles and ligaments. These are known as adhesions. Under most conditions of daily living, the repair job will do well but it may not hold up under a sudden heavy force. The analogy is to a patched tire—safe for travel on a smooth highway but not on a rough rutty road, where the heavy flexing and sudden pressure can work the patch loose.

Aside from the direct mechanical interference with function of an individual muscle or ligament, the patch job in either the prime movers or the vertebral stabilization system can alter the patterns of activity of muscular groups. If an individual with a chronic low back problem sits down for five minutes and then stands up, there may be no difficulty. But if he now sits in the same chair for four hours and then stands up, his back can be both painful and stiff. While it is the quick answer to say that his joints stiffened up, another reason is closer to the truth. The patterns of activity, the timing that tells which muscles when to contract and with how much force, are off. The awareness of the patterns that are "off" comes about in the pain and stiffness. The patterns are not really under direct voluntary control, but they can be strengthened through learning. Then when they are called to action it is with more certainty and strength.

This is a major point of the warm-up for an athletic activity. Most people who believe in the warm-up (there are some trainers who don't!) look upon it as a means of improving the excellence of the performance that follows. But its great point is to forestall the possibility of injury. Almost every action that is performed, whether it is raising a foot or straightening an elbow, demands the activity of more than one muscle. It is not only the strength of a muscle's contraction that is important but also the timing of the activity of one muscle with relation to its neighbor that determines how good or appropriate the final movement or stance will be. In some people the timing, the pattern development, occurs rapidly without the necessity for much training. These are the "naturals." In others, more of a learning process is required. The normal basis for imprinting these patterns is through repetition. This is the point of practice, whether its aim is the hitting of a tennis ball or the running of a mile. The warm-up serves to recall or to reinforce muscular interplay. When a muscle or its attachments have been injured, its timing may be altered. The pattern may require even a greater amount of warm-up to be smooth. A ragged pattern can cause further injury. The action of the exercise program is not only to strengthen the needed muscles but to help strengthen the pattern of their concerted action.

10

Surgery

SURGERY HAS A place in the treatment of low back derangements. It is not, however, a quick and easy, surefire answer. The indications for it must be carefully considered, since spine surgery cannot be looked upon as a minor procedure.

The surgery is approached from two standpoints. The first is to help correct the faulty stabilization, the second is to relieve pressure on a nerve root. The two may be combined in one operation.

In the first type of operation the usual aim is to get a fusion between two vertebrae. Through the application of bone (or bone-stimulating) substance it is hoped that the two vertebrae will fuse together. After fusion they will move as one unit. If the other muscles (such as prime movers) are in spasm in an attempt to stabilize the faulty vertebral unit and are causing back stiffness, the stiffness may decrease after surgery. It may seem paradoxical that an operation to keep two vertebrae from moving results in more flexibility. But the surgery eliminates a source of pain, and when that source is eliminated, the inhibition to move is eliminated. An anology can be found in a broken wrist. The individual will keep the entire extremity still to prevent motion at the wrist.

But if the wrist is immobilized in a cast, the arm and finger can then move with greater freedom.

Other operations are performed to cut down on painful motion between vertebrae. Ends of bone that impinge on each other are removed. Sometimes tight muscles or their covering, the fascia, are cut to loosen abnormal pulls or to restore a balance of power.

Operations to relieve nerve root pressure are called laminectomy and foraminotomy. The laminectomy goes through a portion of the spinal canal to remove an offending disc; the foraminotomy opens the canal through which the nerve root passes on its way out of the spine. Both operations may be performed at one time.

Often there is less than total satisfaction with the results of surgery. When it is done in carefully selected cases and there are no complications such as poor healing, post operative adhesions or abnormal deep scarring, the results tend to be very good. A good deal of the dissatisfaction comes about because of unrealistic hopes that the surgery will yield a completely normal back capable of withstanding all sorts of stress. This does not always happen. Susseccful surgery will yield a better back than before; the percentage of betterment depends on many factors, the most important of which is the restoration of a proper pattern of muscular action with sufficient strength to meet the demands imposed upon it.

11

Treatment

THE TREATMENT FOR the chronic back derangement consists of activities that will improve the action of the muscular apparatus of the back and remove chronic stress or minimize sudden improper stress.

In the activities of daily living it is necessary to use our muscular equipment. It is better for our muscular health to do five units of activity a day for seven days than to do thirty-five units in two hours on a Sunday. One of the aspects of our civilization that works to the detriment of our physical selves is the increasing tendency for energy control. By means of push-buttons large amounts of energy are channeled to take the place of muscular activities. Stairs do not have to be climbed, water does not have to be fetched, and soon pavements will not have to be walked. This is not a plea for a return to the more personal energy requirements of a past time. It is only to point out the fact that the muscular disuse that advancing civilization furthers must be dealt with. Because of the lack of demand for back activity an exercise program will help to fulfill that need. In addition, the exercise program will improve back posture. And by improving the back posture, it is hoped to remove a constant stress on the low back structures.

BACK EXERCISES

Although no two backs are precisely alike, the majority of back derangements share a characteristic mechanical distortion of the proper relationship of the pelvis and sacrum with the lumbar spine. This characteristic distortion is excessive lordosis of the lumbar spine with an increased lumbosacral angle. This results in an increased shearing force on the lumbosacral junction and, to a lesser degree, on the lower lumbar intervertebral spaces. These factors have been described in some detail in Chapter 3.

Because of this characteristic shared by so many faulty backs, the main objective of an exercise program is to improve the relationship of the pelvis and sacrum with the lumbar spine—that is, to flatten out the lumbar lordotic curve and thus relieve the shearing force on the lumbosacral junction and lumbar intervertebral spaces. This improvement in position not only decreases the shearing force on the annulus fibrosus, but relieves the strain on supporting ligaments and positions the muscles so that they are able to exert a better force. The desired position is initiated by tilting the front of the pelvis upward. Such a pelvic tilt is the keystone of the entire exercise program. The pelvic tilt is accomplished primarily by the abdominal muscles, which extend from the rib cage to the front of the pelvis. Tilting the pelvis by actively contracting the abdominal muscles should be accompanied by strong, symmetrical, isometric contraction of all of the muscles of the back and buttocks. Contrary to the usual isotonic, or moving, exercises, isometric exercises are ones in which muscles are contracted and exercised without movement of the parts of the body to which the muscles are attached, and they are an effective method to strengthen and train muscles. Lack of movement is desirable in the presence of painful structures and irritated tissues. For example, a sprained ankle or wrist is put at rest to allow it to heal.

Once the pelvic tilt is mastered, it becomes the starting maneuver for each of the other exercises which prepare the muscles and ligaments of the body for the ultimate goal of the entire program—to stand, sit and move with the pelvis and sacrum in good relationship to the lumbar spine.

The following is a series of six basic exercises designed to maintain or restore the desired mechanical alignment to the spine and the proper interplay of action to the muscles and ligaments of the back. These exercises are designed to correct the mechanical faults which most commonly contribute to derangement of the low back or result from injury to the back. They are useful therapeutically for the majority of faulty backs and as a preventive measure for normal backs. However, it must be realized that some backs will need a modification of this program because of the presence of abnormalities which differ from those which occur most commonly. This difference must be recognized by a physician and prescribed for accordingly. It must also be realized that even a back which may ultimately benefit from these basic exercises may not tolerate them during the acutely painful stage of back derangement. The exercises must be done in a relaxed fashion when the pressure of time is not important. They should not be done when one is very tired, since muscles that are fatigued cannot perform with adequate efficiency and coordination. They should be performed on a hard surface, preferably the floor. When possible the exercises should be preceded by a warm bath or shower or, if more convenient, by the application of a heating pad or other means of heat to the low back. All exercises should be performed slowly— never in a rapid or jerky fashion. The parts of the body should glide smoothly. It is just as important to relax slowly and smoothly from the final position of the exercise as it is to assume the position slowly and smoothly. The exercises should be learned in a progressive fashion in the order in which they are listed. It is essential that the first exercise—the keystone of the entire program—be mastered thoroughly before the second exercise is undertaken. Without instruction by a physical therapist it may take several days or even a week to become proficient in performing the first exercise. When one can perform the exercise well and has sufficient endurance to perform it five times twice a day without pain, then one is ready to progress to the second exercise. Endurance for the second exercise, also, should be increased sufficiently to permit its performance five times twice a day. As further exercises are mastered, the frequency of each exercise should be decreased so that once all of the exercises have been learned properly, each of the exercises should be performed twice in each of two sessions a day. Then gradually, as one's tolerance and muscular strength permit, the repetitions for each exercise should be increased to five times each twice a day.

EXERCISE 1

1. Lie down on the floor face up with hips and knees bent so that your feet are resting on the floor.

2. Press the small of your back hard against the floor and tighten your buttocks and abdominal muscles. This should cause the front part of your pelvis to rotate upward toward your rib cage.

3. Tuck your chin in so as to flatten the back of your neck against the floor.

4. Hold this position for a slow count of five. Do not hold your breath—remember to breathe slowly and freely.

5. Then relax by releasing slowly in this order—neck, shoulders, abdomen and buttocks.

The posture achieved by the spine in this first exercise is the ultimate posture which the spine should learn to maintain. This exercise has further importance in preparing the back and protecting it from pain for the ensuing exercises. There are subtle mistakes which are very easy to make in doing this "keystone" exercise and which

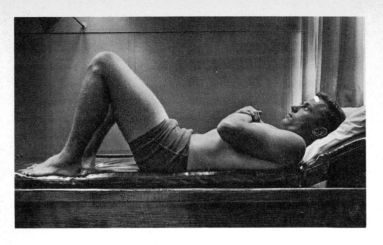

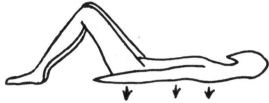

Exercise 1.

will cancel all benefit from doing the exercise and, in fact, can cause increased pain in the low back. It is quite easy for an unskilled person, especially when trying too vigorously to do this exercise, to make the mistake of arching the back off the floor instead of doing exactly the opposite, that is, flattening the small of the back against the floor. It is helpful to have a second person place a hand under the small of the back the first few times to determine whether one is flattening one's back properly against the floor. Another mistake that is often made is to push with the feet to rotate the pelvis upward instead of accomplishing this with the abdominal muscles. When doing each exercise it is important to remember to breathe slowly and freely.

EXERCISE 2

1. Repeat exercise 1 to the hold position.
2. Bend your right hip so that your knee comes toward

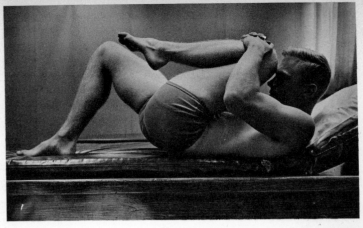

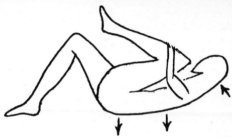

Exercise 2.

your chest. Grasp your knee with both hands and draw it firmly toward your chest.

3. Tuck in your chin and attempt to touch your forehead to your knee. Hold this position for a slow count of five, again remembering to breathe.

4. Slowly return your neck to the starting position and then your knee. Then relax as in exercise 1.

5. Repeat the above steps, bringing your left knee to your chest.

Once the final position of the exercise is achieved, that is, the hip is bent, the knee is pulled toward the chest, and the forehead is touched to the knee, the entire spine has been stretched into a more or less smooth C-curve. This maneuver permits gentle, comfortable stretching of tight ligaments and muscles in the back and hips that may be contributing to pain to the low back.

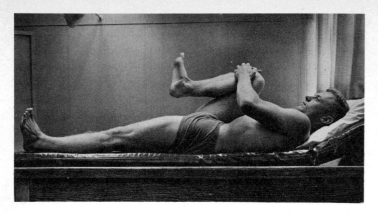

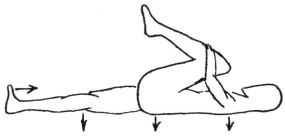

Exercise 3.

1. Again, repeat exercise 1 to the hold position.

2. Bring your right knee to your chest, grasp the knee in both hands and draw the knee firmly to your chest.

3. Slide your left heel down along the floor until your entire left leg is flattened against the floor.

4. Keep your left knee straight. Press the back of your knee firmly against the floor and pull your foot upward so that your toes come toward your shin.

5. Hold for a count of five. Slowly slide your left heel back to the starting position and then return your right leg to the starting position. Then relax as in exercise 1.

6. Repeat the above steps, bringing your left knee to your chest and straightening your right leg against the floor.

The purpose of this exercise is to stretch out and relieve the tightness of the hip flexor muscles, the muscles that bend the thigh forward on the trunk. Why is this important in correcting problems of the low back? If the hip flexor muscles are tight, it becomes impossible to straighten the hips out completely and, therefore, impossible to stand absolutely erect without increasing the lordosis of the lumbar spine. It has already been pointed out that increased lordosis of the lumbar spine is mechanically undesirable for the back and is a great cause of back strain and pain.

It must be emphasized that exercises 1, 2 and 3 must be mastered with maximum proficiency before proceeding to exercises 4, 5 and 6. The latter three exercises are more difficult than the first three and require that the back be well conditioned by the first three exercises. When exercises 1, 2, 3 can be performed well four times each twice a day, then the back is ready for exercise 4.

EXERCISE 4

1. Repeat exercise 1 to the hold position.
2. Straighten your right knee and pull your right foot upward toward your right shin. Then raise your right leg, keeping your knees straight, toward your head. When the leg is raised as far as possible without bending the knee, hold for a count of five and then slowly return the right leg to the starting position. Then relax as in exercise 1.
3. Repeat the above steps, straightening and raising your left leg.

This exercise is designed to loosen tight hamstring muscles, the muscles that extend from the pelvis down the back of the thigh to a point just below the knee joint. Tightness of the hamstring muscles is the usual reason why people cannot bend over and touch the floor without bending their knees; when tight they act as a checkrein on forward bending of the trunk when the knees are kept straight. Tightness in these hamstring muscles is undesirable for the low back because they

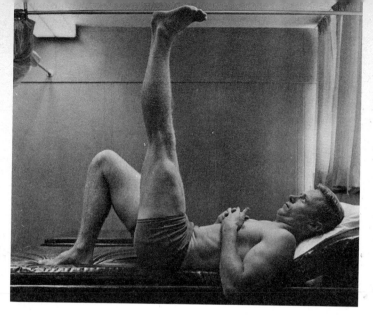

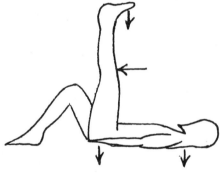

Exercise 4.

demand that more of the bending in leaning over be done in the lumbosacral spine than is normally desirable. Caution must be taken in doing this exercise when one has had a recently ruptured disc or other condition which irritates the sciatic nerve and causes pain to radiate down the leg. In attempting to stretch the hamstring muscles, stress is also placed upon the sciatic nerve and can cause a flare-up of pain in a nerve which is already irritated.

When exercises 1, 2, 3 and 4 can be performed well three times each twice a day, one may proceed to exercise 5.

91

EXERCISE 5

1. Repeat exercise 1 to the hold position.
2. Have another person hold your ankles or feet against the floor or secure your feet under the edge of a couch or other piece of furniture.
3. With both arms reaching forward tuck in your chin and slowly curl up into a sitting position.
4. Hold for a count of five. Then uncurl slowly by allowing your mid-back to reach the floor first, followed by your shoulders, neck and head.
5. Relax as in exercise 1.

Strengthening of the abdominal muscles has already

Exercise 5.

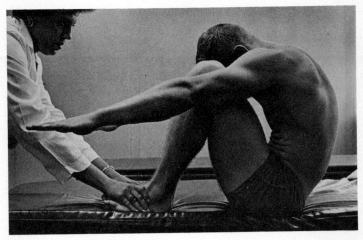

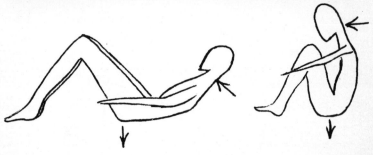

been initiated by contracting them in performing the pelvic tilt. Considerable strengthening can be accomplished with the isometric exercises alone. However, it is desirable to increase the strength of the abdominal muscles as much as possible. The sit-up imposes greater work upon the abdominal muscles and, thereby, contributes to greater strengthening of these muscles. This exercise is not recommended for a person who has sustained a recent compression fracture of a vertebra or who has osteoporosis of the spine.

EXERCISE 6

1. Stand in a doorway with your back against the door frame. Place your heels four inches away from the frame.

Exercise 6.

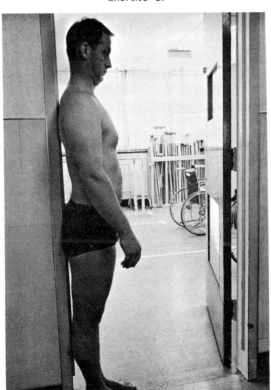

93

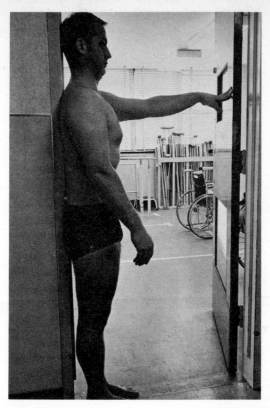

2. Flatten the small of your back against the frame of the door and tighten your buttocks and abdominal muscles, allowing your knees to bend a little. Your pelvis should then be tilted just as it was when you were lying on the floor in exercise 1.

3. Tuck in your chin and flatten your neck against the door frame.

4. For counter-balance reach forward with your arms and press both hands against the opposite side of the door frame.

5. Straighten both knees. At this point the back of your entire neck and trunk is pressing against the door frame.

6. Hold for a count of five and then relax.

This is the final exercise in the six basic exercises and must not be done until the first five exercises are completely mastered. It is the final exercise which prepares the spine to assume the proper posture when sitting, standing and walking. When mastered successfully, it should condition the spine so well that it automatically assumes and maintains the right posture.

Certain precautions have been emphasized in the preliminary discussion of the exercise program and in the discussion following certain of the individual exercises. Warning must be given to anyone who attempts to undertake this exercise program on his own. If any exercise produces pain, particularly while it is being performed or even within a period of twelve to twenty-four hours following performance of the exercise, something is wrong. Of course, if the pain is delayed for several hours after doing the exercise, it may be due to other intervening activities which imposed a stress upon the back. The pain also may be due to the incorrect performance of one or more of the exercises. Usually, if the pelvic tilt is mastered well, the lumbosacral spine is then protected well in each of the other exercises. Certain small mistakes which are frequently responsible for incorrect performance of the pelvic tilt are described under Exercise 1. Pain may also result if the exercises are attempted too soon after an acute episode of severe back derangement. And, as already indicated, a certain few backs have mechanical abnormalities that will not benefit from these specific exercises and, perhaps, will not even tolerate them. It is to be expected that many individuals for whose backs these exercises are suited will experience discomfort during the first few days of performing the exercises, but this discomfort should be only that of muscular soreness such as one experiences after the first tennis game of the season or working in the garden for the first time in the spring. If there is a recurrence of or increase in low back pain or radiating pain upon doing the exercises, the exercises should be discontinued until further medical advice can be obtained. Many patients will require the instruction and discipline of a physical therapist, under the prescription of a physician, in order to master the exercises properly and to have effective carry-over of proper posture and function in daily activities.

The mere performance of a few exercises once or even twice a day with disregard for the posture or use of the back for the remainder of the day will do little to correct a malfunctioning back. The exercises should be regarded as basic training to prepare the back to function in a mechanically satisfactory manner during the day's activities. The average person engages in various physical activities, many of which may impose stress upon his low back. In fact, many low backs are under fairly constant stress throughout a twenty-four hour day. Treatment of a chronic low back derangement can be effective only if the stress imposed upon the structures of the low back by the activities of daily living are removed. Certain activities must be given special consideration. The patient with a low back problem must know if a certain activity can be done, at what stage should it be tried, and if there is a special way of doing it.

WALKING

One of the most useful of daily activities is walking. Anyone touched with the slightest suspicion of a low back difficulty should seize any opportunity to walk. If the individual is just starting his rehabilitation, the walking should be gradually increased to a least one mile a day. The walk should be brisk. The human frame is not well adapted to plain standing. It is a common experience to become quickly fatigued when walking slowly with frequent standing, as in window shopping. If the same distance were covered in a well-paced walk, much less fatigue would result. As the tolerance to the distance and gait improve, and if the social circumstances permit, the walk can be converted into a jog. This form of gait puts more stress on the back and so is useful in the later stages of rehabilitation. Walking should not be confined to level ground; using stairs for brief transits is a good idea. It has seemed to the writer that, with the automation of the passenger elevator, one has no shorter wait than twenty-five years ago, and walking may help dispel some of that ever-increasing aspect of our existence—tension. Anyone with low back difficulty is well rid of that element.

Naturally the subject of walking brings up shoes. There is only one thing to be said about shoes: They should be comfortable. A badly fitting shoe can cause a hobbled gait which can produce unwelcome back stress by not permitting a full free swing through on each step. Many physicians suffer from the belief that the only good shoes are low heels or flats. Heels serve a purpose in walking. If the walking surface is hard and unyielding a tough sole is necessary to protect the bottom of the foot. Such a firm sole interferes with the action of the toes in the push off. The heel compensates for the externally forced mechanical disadvantage of the rigid sole. This fact was discovered by the Roman Legionnaires a long time ago.

For running, a heel is not necessary and, in certain sports, a heel interferes with the action of the foot and so blocks a spring-like flexibility. Many women, through long use of heels and avoidance of certain sports, have a shortening of the calf muscles and tendons. Often back aches can be induced in this group by having them switch to low heels. It is then possible to relieve back ache by switching them back to a higher heel. This is all by way of a preface to the point that a medium height heel may be the best for walking. And this applies to both sexes. A person who suddenly decreases his heel height and is on his feet a great deal may experience such fatigue by the end of the day that he is disinclined to do any walking. Very often the reason is not apparent to the patient.

A point should be made about certain painful foot conditions. It is possible to have a low back derangement with backache only and a separate or unrelated foot disability that gives rise to severe pain, even a sciatic radiation. The two conditions are unrelated, but the doctor and the patient may integrate both conditions into one ailment, and the patient may be saddled with a diagnosis of a low back derangement with nerve root pressure caused by a herniated lumbar disc. The shoes picked for walking, or, for that matter, normal activities, should not foster any disturbing foot conditions. Certain shoe corrections or supports may be necessary to relieve painful foot complaints.

Another element concerning shoes should be mentioned here. Certain individuals have unequal leg lengths. This demands an additional increase in mobility of the back with each step, and so increases the wear and tear on the back. Though this may be tolerated for a long time, eventually the straw that is always breaking the camel's back may cause too much of a strain. The result is that there may be a prolonged disability based on the continuing stress caused by the difference in leg length. In many such cases the use of a raised heel to compensate for the difference may produce marked relief for the patient.

TRAVELING AND DRIVING

It has been mentioned before that an activity to which a back does not take kindly is the prolonged maintenance of one position. This applies to other muscular systems, not just those of the low back. A fixed position held for a long time can bother a perfectly normal back as well as one that has a derangement. Many of today's airplane seats cause long-range discomfort. The compromise between allowable space and an attempt to get the appearance of easeful reclining has resulted in forcing the traveler into an unnaturally flexed position with too much weight on the base of his spine. In addition, the attempt to get to a standing posture from that position demands a thrusting forward of the trunk which can cause an extra strain. The old-fashioned train seat that was short seated and straight backed and forced the traveler to stretch his legs by walking around in a swaying car led to more generalized fatigue but less lasting back discomfort.

Most modern automobile seats seem to have a common parentage with the airplane seat. On a long trip, the passengers have the advantage of being able to move about on their seats (within the limits of their safety harnesses), but the driver is constrained to keep his position. To overcome this difficulty and to help maintain bodily fitness, the driver should stop driving for five minutes out of every hour and should walk around to release accumulated tension and get his muscles acting again. He should be careful that his seat permits a good upright posture. His weight should be distributed on both thighs and buttocks. He should not be forced into a jack-knifed position with extended legs. The seat should not be so soft that he is engulfed. There should be some squirming room. A bad seat will not only interfere with pedal action but also cause back strain while switching from brake to gas.

SITTING AND SEATS

While the individual with a normal back has a wide range of sitting positions and seats that can be tolerated, the patient with a low back disability is much more limited. A good seat should be, roughly, the height of the knee above the floor. A person sitting in such a seat will have his knees at a right angle while his soles and heels can be placed in contact with the floor. The seat itself should not be longer than the distance from the back of the calf to the back of the buttocks. If it is too long, then on sitting down the back has to go backward into a hyperextended position. This is an awkward position for a deranged back. The back of the chair should offer support from the region of, at least, the lower third of the rib cage down to the sacrum.

When a person wants to maintain an erect position his center of gravity must be over his feet or else he will topple. The center of gravity is in the middle of the lower half of the body, so this point must be over the feet. When a person rises from the seated position the center of gravity has to be arched forward and up. If the feet are forward then the center of gravity has to be moved forward. But if the feet can be placed under the seat then the center of gravity does not have to be propelled so far forward. The stuffed armchair, whose front edge comes down to the floor, will not permit the feet to be placed back under the seat. If the chair is low and there is no hand rest to help in the elevation then the back requires forceful stabilization and a heavy muscular motion to get the center of gravity where it belongs. The automobile seat offers special difficulties in this regard. The driver not only has to lever himself forward but more to the left. The more modern, low cars demand greater trunk action than did the older cars with their higher seats.

RESTING AND SLEEPING

The period given up to sleep serves a special purpose from the psychological viewpoint. It is the time when the relevant portion of the day's activities are fitted into the individual's experience structure. On the physical level it gives the body's tissues a chance to repair the effects of the day's trauma. The body and particularly the low back should rest in the most favorable position. For the back the most favorable position, the one that imposes the least strain, is a straightened position of the spine. In this position there is neither much flexion or extension. For every joint in the body there is a "rest" position. This is as much true of a finger or elbow joint as it is of the

100

back. If a joint is immobilized, as in a plaster cast, in a position other than the rest position, the joint is strained through overstretching of the ligaments. After removal of the cast there will be excessive stiffness.

The rest position of the spine resembles that seen in the pre-walking infant. The resting surface should not prevent one from assuming that posture. A point to be remembered is that a great deal of motion takes place during sleep in most normal individuals. Unless drugged or over-fatigued they twist and turn in varying degrees. The movements are below the conscious level, as is the awareness to move back from the edge of the bed to prevent a fall. If the mattress is very soft, turning to a new position requires more force and stiffening of the back than if it is firm and offers resistance. A firm mattress demands less work and less rigid back stabilization. Although it might seem paradoxical, a more restful sleep will be obtained from such a surface than from a soft mattress.

It is possible to have a firm surface that curves. If the curve is too low in the middle or at either end it will throw the back into straining postures either on side or back resting positions. Only two choices are mentioned, because lying face down—"stomach sleeping"—is a strain on a bad back (also on a bad neck). The position throws the back into an extended, strained position. It is necessary to turn the head to a marked sideways position in order to breathe. This can similarly strain the ligaments of the upper spine.

To avoid the curved mattress, a bed board is frequently prescribed. The bed board should be of sufficient stiffness to prevent a sag in the middle of the bed. For the average person it should be from $\frac{1}{2}$- to $\frac{3}{4}$-inch plywood; a lesser thickness permits the middle dip. The usefulness of the bedboard can be checked prior to purchase if the patient puts the mattress on the floor for three or four nights. If the mattress is too soft and thin the individual's boney

101

prominences will be under too much pressure. A restless night will result as the individual tries to avoid the painful pressure points.

LIFTING

Lifting objects is a common factor in triggering back pain. The person who does a lot of lifting regularly, whose muscles are in good shape and who knows the proper way to lift rarely gets a bad back from lifting. But the business executive, the sedentary office worker, the housewife, all of whom lift infrequently, whose muscles are in poor shape and who do not know how to lift properly—these are the people who will hurt their back with lifting. Typically a bad back may result in these individuals from moving a heavy piece of furniture at home, helping a friend to lift a heavy boat out of the water on a holiday weekend, or even bending over the wrong way and lifting no more than a shoe from the floor. Certainly the person with a history of back trouble is a likely candidate for recurrence of trouble from improper lifting. Such a person should avoid heavy lifting.

When lifting is to be done—by back sufferers or non-back sufferers—it should be done properly even if the object to be picked up is no more than an article of clothing. One should never bend forward or sideways from the waist. The back should be maintained as a straight, upright column, and the bending should be done by the knees. The body is then raised back up by straightening the knees and hips, thus making the legs do the work, not the back.

Individuals with back problems should be equally careful when lifting their own weight out of bed. One should never come directly up to a sitting position from a back-lying position. Instead, one should roll over onto one side, swing the legs over the edge of the bed and then, by pushing with the hands against the surface of the bed, raise the trunk up sideways to a sitting position.

102

SPORTS

In the world of today sports play a more prominent role in the lives of more and more people. Increased leisure time, better transportation, improved media of communication and many other factors have contributed to a progressively greater participation in many sports. As the number of people from the general population interested in sports increases, the number of people with bad backs interested in sports increases.

Before considering specific sports, attention must be directed to certain general principles. As mentioned earlier, the warm-up is very important for all individuals participating in a sport, but especially for those with a bad back. Professional athletes always warm up before their actual performance in a game. The warm-up may be the deciding factor as to whether a bad back will tolerate a sport or not. There are several differences to be noted between the expert athlete and the unskilled amateur. The expert is in good physical condition with trained muscles and engages in his sport regularly. The unskilled athlete, frequently in poor muscular condition, may participate in primarily sedentary activities throughout the week and engage in a sport only on weekends or even less frequently. The better muscular condition and greater athletic skill of the expert enables him to protect himself from injury with greater success than the unskilled athlete.

What sports are compatible with a bad back? The answer is "not many" if the back has been recently painful. The best sports for the individual with a chronic back are swimming and hiking. However, even swimming must be done with certain restrictions when it is first attempted after an episode of low back pain. Before any swimming should be done, the back should be well along on a program of reconditioning with the exercises already described and with gradually increasing amounts of walking. When swimming is first begun, the strokes should be limited to only two—floating on one's back with kicking of the legs and paddling of the hands to either side of the trunk, and a side stroke. Both of these strokes keep the spine slightly flexed so that it will not be subjected to the stress of hyperextension. Later, when one has trained one's muscles and built up a tolerance for exercise, other strokes may be attempted very carefully. Diving should not be done.

As already discussed earlier, walking is excellent for the back. Therefore, hiking is a sport compatible with a bad back, once the back has improved to a non-painful stage and re-conditioning has been accomplished through exercises. When first undertaken after an acute episode of back pain, hiking should be limited to smooth terrain and short distances. Later, as the tolerance of the back permits, somewhat more rugged terrain and longer distances may be attempted.

What can be said for other, more demanding sports? By virtue of its popularity golf must be given consideration. Of course, the walking involved in golf is good for the back—provided the player is not carrying his own golf bag. Riding in a golf cart eliminates the benefit of the walking and may, in fact, be detrimental to the back because of the sitting and the unpredictable jostling of the cart. The golf stroke, itself, imposes a twisting, shearing action of the low back that is undesirable. The degree of twisting varies with the form used. Some chronically deranged low backs will tolerate golf reasonably well, others will not. Once the back has been adequately re-conditioned with exercises and walking and no pain has been experienced for several months, it may be safe to resume golf cautiously. The decision to play golf must be left up to the judgment of the patient, perhaps with the help of advice from his physician.

Tennis is an even more demanding sport than golf in that it imposes a greater stress on the low back. There is a greater twisting, shearing action in the lumbosacral spine which is more forceful than that involved in golf and occurs frequently in an abrupt, unexpected fashion. Also, particularly in the serve, there is frequently a forceful hyperextension of the lumbosacral spine. Most low backs with chronic derangement will not tolerate tennis.

Handball, squash and other racquet sports impose stresses similar to those of tennis, although perhaps not as forceful. These sports, also, are probably best avoided by the individual with a bad back.

Bowling has become a popular sport. Depending on the form used, it may be tolerated by the chronically deranged back, but certainly only after the back has been well reconditioned by exercises and walking. The dangers of bowling lie in the possibilities of causing too much strain to one side in picking up and carrying the ball and of hyperextending the lumbosacral spine upon releasing the ball.

What about skiing? Skiing an ordinary, straight, smooth downhill course would seem to impose relatively little dangerous stress on the low back—in fact, the posture of the back under those skiing circumstances is mechanically good for the back. However, one cannot always count on a smooth, straight downhill course; abrupt turns and spills are almost inevitable for the average skier. And certainly the slalom and other maneuvers impose undesirable strain upon the low back.

Water skiing is out of the question for the chronically deranged low back. The technique of water skiing demands that the lumbosacral spine be maintained in considerable hyperextension. In addition, the danger of falling imposes further risk of injury to the back.

12

Sex and the
Aching Back

IT HAS BEEN the author's experience that most physicians
shy away from discussing the subject of sexual activity
and low back derangement. Many think it is too complex
a problem. Perhaps even more significant is an unstated
feeling that the psychological factors are important
but so difficult to grasp or to manage that they would
just as soon not get involved. Its role in disability demands some exposition of the subject.

When there is an acute low back derangement, fracture or other severe condition, any motion of the lower
trunk or pelvis will be painful. The afflicted partner
probably cannot do any structural damage by the induced
movement. The "cease and desist" orders coming from
the pain awareness center will effectively limit activity
before damage is done. It is extremely doubtful, except
in rather unusual circumstances, that the permitted body
exertions can surmount the pain enough to allow passion
to have its full expression.

As the acute stage is generally limited in time, either
subsiding by itself or with treatment, the problem of
long-range satisfactory sexual expression is not serious.
All that is demanded is either patience or adaptability.
If the attacks occur often with shorter trouble-free in-

tervals between, then more rigorous back treatment is needed to minimize the emotional consequences or disability imposed by the back. The significant interrelationship, then, is between the chronic low back derangement and sexual activity. The major questions that confront the treating physician are (1) is there a disturbance in libido and/or performance and (2) can sexual activities do damage?

If the physician is to help the patient he must tread very carefully when considering the first question. He must decide, by careful enquiry, if fear of inducing pain is having a serious inhibiting effect. Under normal conditions—or more properly, in individuals who are reacting normally—the fear reaction can effectively squelch the response to stimuli that normally would excite. Both the emotional and physical exhibitions that constitute the response will be lacking. This state of affairs can be helped by reassurance, guidance and both physical and medical treatment.

If the back difficulty is being used as a means of withdrawal from an undesirable situation, the outlook is not as hopeful. The use of a physical disability to accomplish this end is not necessarily a willful act on the part of the patient. For reasons beyond the scope of this discussion, a feeling of sexual inadequacy or lack of sexual interest may arise in the behavioral environment of the patient. In our modern terminology, the channels of communication no longer function well or the contents and boundaries of the domain are too well known to be of interest. This can happen in a marital as well as an extramarital relationship.

Though it is more pronounced with advancing age, no sexually active age group is immune to this withdrawal. The need for preservation of the self-image cannot permit a poor response. The bad back offers the refuge—the explanation to both the inside and outside worlds. Of course, there may be other than the sexual basis for withdrawal from an unpleasant situation. But no matter what is at the base of the situation, treatment directed towards the back alone will not solve the problem nor outwardly help the back to any extent. An attempt to help the patient by showing that his back problem is an excuse will usually not work well. The frank exposition of the condition can further wound the already suffering self-image. All connected with the problem—the physician, well-intentioned, analytical friends—may feel the full force of the patient's resentment if his (or her) motivation is brought forth. The net result may be a relapse into a more intense disability.

The next aspect is whether the sexual act can do harm to the back. It is assumed, for this discussion, that there is no detriment or bar to the act, that its performance, aside from the present physical consideration, is not overlaid with tenseness or any unhappy emotional aura. Also, the act does not drain either partner of any of life's energy supply, weaken the spiritual force or sap the strength. The very normal post-coital overactivity in the female and languor to sleepiness in the male do not, for either sex, mean an unhappy or unsatisfied physical state. Our discussion will be concerned with the normal body positioning. It is understood that geography can alter the meaning of the word "normal"; in this we are using the relatively unsophisticated Western Hemispheres (English-speaking) standard positioning. The natural body attitude and motions bear a strong tie-in to the exercise program.

In the program, the constant emphasis has been on the relationship between the pelvis and the lumbar spine. The main purpose of the training is to bring the pelvis into line with the spine. The resulting decrease in lumbosacral angle relieves the shearing force on the lumbosacral junction. This keeps the supporting ligaments from being in a state of constant strain and enables the muscles to be in a position where they can exert better force. The desired position occurs when the front of the pelvis tilts upwards. The chief muscles for the tilt are the gluteal muscles in the buttocks and the lower abdominal muscles. If the individual stands with his (her) back against a wall, normally, the contact with the surface is near the shoulder blades and at the buttocks. In between these points is a hollow formed between the lumbo-sacral region and the wall. A hand can be placed in this hollow. The aim of our treatment is to eliminate this space. The proper pelvic tilt will do it. The upward tilting of the pelvis shifts the lumbo-sacral region backward. This is accomplished by forceful contraction of the gluteal and lower abdominal muscles. If the resulting motion is observed, it will be seen that this results in a pelvic thrust, the basic pelvic action in intercourse. The thrust activity has long been considered as a basis for evaluating interested response in both male and female. The musculature of significance for sexual activity is the same set of muscles that are the object of attention in the low back exercises.

There are two stories that are relevant here. The first is literary and perhaps actually happened. It is found in the *Autobiography of Frank Harris.* Harris states that he deliberately exercised in order to strengthen his activity during sexual intercourse. He thought that horseback riding was particularly useful. Actually, maintaining a proper seat for some gaits does demand a great deal of abdominal and gluteal muscular action.

The second is an authenticated story that concerns a patient who wound up under police scrutiny. Her doctor was a strong proponent of the low back flexion exercise. The young lady, who had just received instruction in the movement, was waiting in the street for a bus. As she stood there, she went through the motions to help fix them in her mind. The well-intentioned pelvic thrusts, known popularly as "bumps," brought the police.

It is possible, by lower extremity positioning or position alteration, to avoid an over-extended position of the back for the sexual participant. In this connection, the firm mattress is an aid to pelvic flexion or proper tilt.

A bed that is too soft allows the buttocks to sink down too far and throw the back into an unfavorable position.

If all the symptoms and signs are caused by a chronic low back derangement, then there is no physical reason to inhibit or limit sexual activity. It does happen, however, in some conditions, that there is constriction of nerves in the lower abdominal wall, sometimes associated with back pain. Sexual activity may accentuate this pain but should not cause any structural damage. Care must be taken not to infer a psychological or emotional causation to the effects produced by this condition.

GLOSSARY

ANTERIOR—Front.

ARTICULATE—Joins with. An articulation is a joint.

AUTONOMIC—That portion of the nervous system that helps to control heart rate, sweating, blood pressure, and other bodily activities not under direct voluntary control.

BILATERAL—Both sides.

CAPSULE—The fibrous sac that encloses a joint. The closed sac maintains a small amount of joint fluid between the surfaces.

CENTRAL NERVOUS SYSTEM—The brain and spinal cord. Abbreviation: C.N.S.

CONGENITAL—A condition present at birth, even though its effects may not be known until later in life.

DISC—The structure that occupies the space between two vertebral bodies. It consists of a tough gelatinous center (the nucleus pulposus) and a surrounding fibrous, ring-shaped structure (the annulus fibrosus).

DURAL SAC—A fibrous membrane that surrounds the central nervous system. It contains the nerve tissue, its covering (the meninges), and the cerebro-spinal fluid.

EDEMA—Swelling of a part of the body caused by an accumulation of fluid within the tissues. The fluid in the main is derived from the liquid part of the blood.

FORAMEN—Hole; opening.

FRACTURE—Break. (Contrary to lay opinion, a fractured bone is the same as a broken bone.)

HORMONE—A substance secreted into the blood stream by certain glands which can affect the growth, development, and condition of other tissues. Such glands are the thyroid, ovary, and adrenals.

INVOLUNTARY—Not under willed or conscious control.

ISOMETRIC—Refers to a muscle contraction in which there is an increase in the force exerted but very little change in length of the muscle.

ISOTONIC—Refers to a muscle contraction in which there is shortening of the muscle or movement with very little change in the force exerted.

111

JOINT—The structure formed where two bones move in contact with each other.

KYPHOSIS—A description of a spine curvature that goes backward, causing the patient to lean forward.

LIGAMENT—Tough fibro-elastic tissue that ties bones together. Unlike a muscle, it has no contractile power.

LORDOSIS—A description of a spine curvature that goes forward. In the low back it corresponds to a sway back.

LUMBAGO—A descriptive term for low back pain. It does not state what is causing the pain.

LUMB-SACRAL—The point of junction between the last lumbar vertebra and the sacrum.

OBJECTIVE—A finding that can be observed by someone other than the experiencing party. Example: a deformity of the foot.

PERIPHERAL NERVE—A nerve that lies beyond the spinal canal. It may carry messages to or away from the C.N.S.

POSTERIOR—Toward the back.

PROGNOSIS—The expected outcome.

REFLEX (as used herein)—An involuntary reaction (usually muscular) caused by a suddenly applied external stimulus. As the connections for the "to" and "from" nerves do not extend across many levels in the C.N.S., or use many pathways, a reflex is often used as a pathway or level indicator.

ROOT—The prolongation and differentiation by level of the spinal cord. The roots on leaving the spinal canal form the peripheral nerves.

RUPTURE—Tear, or break, usually of an enclosure that is holding a material.

SCIATICA—Pain radiating from buttock down the back of the thigh and into the leg. A descriptive term which does not indicate the cause of the pain.

TRAUMA—An injury.

TRAUMATIC—Injurious.

VERTEBRA—One unit of the spine. Plural: vertebrae. Adjective: vertebral.

VOLUNTARY—Under direct control.

VOLUNTARY MUSCLES—Those muscles that are willed, to contract, such as the arm muscles. Muscles of the bowel or of the heart are not under direct voluntary control, and are therefore involuntary muscles.